TOUGH
TALK
ABOUT FAT!

How to Reach and Maintain Your Ideal Weight

William B. Parsons Jr., M.D.

Lilac Press
Scottsdale, Arizona

Although the author and publisher have exhaustively researched many sources to assure the accuracy and completeness of the information contained in this book, we assume no responsibility for errors, inaccuracies, omissions, or other inconsistency herein. Any slights against people or organizations are unintentional.

For further information about this book and *Cholesterol Control Without Diet! The Niacin Solution,*

First printing 2003

ISBN 0-9662568-9-1
LCCN 2003091599

ATTENTION DOCTORS' OFFICES, EMPLOYERS, CORPORATIONS, UNIVERSITIES, COLLEGES, & PROFESSIONAL ORGANIZATIONS:
Quantity discounts are available on bulk purchases of this book for educational purposes. Special books or book excerpts can also be created to fit specific needs. For information, please contact Lilac Press, P.O. Box 1356, Scottsdale, AZ 85252-1356, phone (408) 991-0576.

ACKNOWLEDGEMENTS

The author gratefully acknowledges the following invaluable assistance:

Carey Hindall for library assistance

Christopher O'Brien for computer consultation and the new website

My son, Tyler, for computer guidance and the original website

My wonderful wife, Lynn, for proofreading and helpful comments and for allowing her patience to be tested once again by my time-consuming writing of another book

DEDICATION

To you, the reader, with weight to lose—
whether it is 10 pounds, 100 pounds, or more.

May you use these lessons to
reach and maintain your ideal weight,
look better and feel better,
prevent heart attack and diabetes,
keep from ruining weight-bearing joints,
and improve your quality of life.

Stay well and enjoy every day!

CONTENTS

TABLES AND FIGURE

Introduction

Why another book about weight control? Near the end of 2002, under the heading "Diet," *Books in Print* listed *4,291* titles! And yet the Epidemic of Obesity rages out of control in US. *The Surgeon General's Call to Action to Prevent and Decrease Overweight and Obesity 2001* told us that more than 61% of adults in US are either overweight (30%) or obese (31%). *Obese* means more than 30% over ideal weight. In addition, nearly 13% of American children are obese. All of these figures are much higher than 10 years ago and by now are even higher than just quoted.

Why is this important? Not only because being fat looks bad and reduces quality of life, but for important health reasons as well. We'll emphasize health but won't forget the "look better and feel better" reason for weight control. Obesity increases the risk of heart attack, high blood pressure, and diabetes. It wears out weight-bearing joints. One group estimated that 300,000 Americans die each year from illnesses caused or worsened by obesity.

Researchers in 2002 reported that people overweight at 40 are likely to die at least three years sooner than those who are slim and trim. In terms of life expectancy, being fat at age 40 or beyond is just as bad as smoking. At the present rate, obesity will soon pass smoking as the leading preventable cause of death. Non-smokers classified as overweight but not obese lost an average of three years of life. Obese people died even sooner. Losing excess weight and keeping it off can improve this.

We hasten to add this: *Tough Talk About Fat!* does not scold people for being too heavy. Instead, it urges them to *get tough* with that extra fat and *get rid of it—all of it*, then stay trim. We hope that you will buy several copies of the book for friends and relatives who need it, while encouraging them to do the same for others. We (and you) don't want your gift to seem to say, "You're fat. Here's a book." For this reason, every copy includes a bookmark that explains your concerns and softens the message.

Tough Talk About Fat! is an expanded update of a booklet on weight reduction that I wrote for my internal medicine practice in Scottsdale, Arizona from 1978 until my retirement in 1999. Before 1978, I had always had the luxury of working with dietitians, who instructed patients. During my training years at the Mayo Clinic, we had a superb staff of dietitians. At the Jackson Clinic in Madison, Wisconsin (1956-1974), where I did most of my pioneer research on the first successful drug for cholesterol control (niacin), Mary Hulder and then Ellyn Satter skillfully taught my patients. (More of Ellyn's work and books later.)

Our aim for every patient has always been to *Reach and Maintain Your Ideal Weight*—hence the subtitle. As the Epidemic steadily increases, this goal has become urgent for more people.

My 1998 hardcover book, *Cholesterol Control Without Diet! The Niacin Solution,* summarized in plain words my decades of research and practice in that field. In 2003 we published an expanded, updated second edition in paperback. That book again tells the truth about cholesterol control, why diet fails, and that the widely advertised statin drugs not only lack niacin's distinctive advantages but also have little-known hazards.

In one major development between 1998 and 2003, *obesity* was upgraded to a *major risk factor for heart attack,* rather than a lesser one. Before leaving his position of US Surgeon General at the end of 2001, David Satcher, MD, issued a devastating report about the US Epidemic of Obesity. It stated that 61% of Americans are now overweight, with 30% of them obese (at least 30% above ideal weight). In the previous ten years, the obese segment of the US population had increased from 20% to more than 30%. This trend must be reversed! Everyone needs to take *The Surgeon General's Call to Action to Prevent and Decrease Overweight and Obesity 2001** very seriously.

Why is the Obesity Epidemic progressing at such a pace? Not for lack of reading material! The Satcher report lists 37

**The Surgeon General's Call to Action to Prevent and Decrease Overweight and Obesity 2001.* U.S. Department of Health and Human Services

government books and web sites with information on this topic. Bookstores are full of books with various approaches to excessive weight. This vast array of books obviously has not stemmed the tide of increasing obesity. *Many people in the obese segment of the American public do not buy and read books.* (We'll try later to address this.) Readers can't be sure how much to believe of what they see in newspapers and magazines and can be confused by its apparently complexity. Available books tend to put off the reader with their bickering: more protein, less carbohydrate; more carbohydrate, less protein; more fat, more protein; less fat—on and on.

I decided that our overweight world needs a book that tells briefly and clearly *the truth about weight control* in the same readable, easily understood style that *CCWD!* uses to explain the truth about cholesterol control. This book is the result. It is a revision of my earlier office booklet, but this time we urge people to *get tough with their fat* and *keep up that toughness* every day, every month, every year—to reach and maintain ideal weight.

In the second edition of *CCWD!* we mentioned this book because many persons (or families) who need to control cholesterol also need weight control. But these are two distinct and separate goals. They should not be thought of as one and the same.

The best way to manage problems with the *cholesterol* profile (bad cholesterol and good cholesterol, as well as some finer details) is to *change the body factory.* This requires medication. On the other hand, *the **only** way to lose excessive weight* is to **control calories** in your daily eating.

My aim is to keep the book simple and short. Keeping it simple is easy, because the truth about weight control is not complicated, even though parts may surprise you. Realizing that many people who will not tackle a long book will read a shorter one, I have kept this one as short as possible, while including all the strategies I believe will help you to succeed.

This book will not contain recipes. For years I have noticed, in books on weight control or cholesterol control, that when an author runs out of things to say, he prints recipes. For the same reason, we will not print a detailed calorie table. However, I will direct you to one, a very useful book I would (and did) buy. To make it easier, I will do some of the homework for you, showing you how to get much information with little effort.

As in *CCWD!* I won't say "he/she" each time I use a pronoun that could refer to either sex. Likewise, I will not make this manuscript gender-neutral by changing such pronouns to "persons," "people," or "individuals" in every instance. To resolve the thorny gender issue (although I can't understand why anyone finds it a problem), I will arbitrarily try to refer to a patient as "she" or "her" and a physician as "he" or "him." This is realistic for a couple of reasons. Women are better about going to doctors and taking care of their health than are men, who often wait until a heart attack gets their attention. There still are more men than women doctors, although medical school classes are now about equally divided and the numbers of women in medicine are steadily increasing. I hope my gender decision will not offend anyone or distract any reader from the book's important message.

Now back to work. Get ready to *get tough with your fat.* Don't be offended when I say this to you. It is a matter of life or death, of avoiding serious disability with aging, of looking and feeling good, and of being a role model for children, rather than becoming part of the Obesity Epidemic, with its dire consequences. You must be ready to, as they say in the USMC, "Be a Marine!" or, as we say in the West, "Cowboy up!"

Use the brain and the willpower the good Lord gave you. *Learn how* to get tough with your fat. You must *take charge of your life and of your body. No one else can or will do it for you.* Are you up to the challenge of reaching and maintaining your ideal weight? I can show you how, but *you must do it.*

Are you ready? Let's go!

Do You Really Want to Lose Weight?

Of course you do, or you wouldn't be reading this. Then start out by being sure you understand your reasons for losing weight. Here's my list. See whether it contains your main reason(s); see also whether it contains reasons you hadn't thought about.

1. By losing weight, you will *look and feel better.* This alone should be ample reason to reach and maintain your ideal weight, but there's much, much more.

2. Reducing excess weight will *lower your risk of heart attack, stroke, and death* in a number of ways.

3. Carrying excess weight for years results in *wearing out your weight-bearing joints,* leaving you with the painful consequences of *degenerative joint disease.*

4. *Do not* consider weight reduction as a means to *control cholesterol.* It doesn't work and can do some bad things. I'll explain later.

5. Losing your excessive fat can *help others around you—* particularly your children—to get a grip on their weight problems, thus improving their lives.

Look and feel better. If this is your motivation for getting tough with your fat, I am with you 100%. Why do you suppose weight-losing plans advertise by showing the old, fat pictures and contrasting them with the successful client's more recent, slimmer figure? For many people (perhaps most), their personal appearance is the number one reason for wanting to lose weight. Whether this is your top reason or not, let's use it to help you.

By the way, I recently heard a knowledgeable person state that the weight-reduction industry in the US is a $58 billion a year business with a 98% failure rate! I believe it, and so should you. In his syndicated column, George Will said that "Americans spend more than $30 billion a year on weight-loss products and programs." Now there's quite a difference between those figures on dollars spent. Both amounts are beyond my comprehension.

The important figure is the overwhelming failure rate! But *you* are going to succeed. The success rate of persons who use the information in this book properly and persistently will be much, much higher than 2%. In fact, it will be 100%. Any deviation from this ideal will be because of an individual's failure to learn these teachings and apply them consistently. Don't be that person!

Do you have a recent photograph? Maybe not; fat people often don't like to have pictures taken. One of the ways to gauge your progress will be how you look. We need a starting point. If you don't have a recent photo, take at least two pictures, date them, and put them in the front of your weight loss diary. One should be in normal clothing, to show how large you are and what you are wearing to try to look thinner. The other should be in a bathing suit (if you have one that fits) or in underwear. You aren't going to put these photos in *People* magazine or on a pornographic web site; they are just for you to compare in six months and at whatever other intervals you choose. As you progress, they will confirm how much better you look, even as your friends notice the change and compliment you about it.

Reduce your risk of heart attack, stroke, diabetes, and death. *The Surgeon General's Call to Action* says that our approach should focus on health rather than appearance, and he's right. Excess weight increases your risk of high blood pressure and diabetes. Both of these increase your chance of heart attack or stroke. And these, in turn, result in death or serious disability.

Do you need figures to convince you? American Heart Association (AHA) estimates say that each year more than 300,000 Americans die of causes related to obesity. Who are these obese persons, many of whom will die of this correctable disorder?

Table 1 shows the breakdown by age and ethnic group. But regardless of where you stand in regard to the national figures, let's say that there's only one important overweight person—*you.*

Table 1

Overweight and Obesity in US, by Age and Ethnic Groups

Overweight Children, 6-11	Boys	Girls
Non-Hispanic whites	10.3%	9.2%
Non-Hispanic blacks	11.9%	16.4%
Mexican-Americans	17.4%	14.3%

Overweight Adolescents, 12-17	Boys	Girls
Non-Hispanic whites	11.1%	8.5%
Non-Hispanic blacks	10.7%	15.7%
Mexican-Americans	14.6%	13.7%

Overweight* Americans, 18 and Older	Men	Women
Non-Hispanic whites	62.4%	43.0%
Non-Hispanic blacks	64.1%	64.5%
Hispanics	64.7%	56.8%
Non-Hispanic Asian-Pacific Islanders	35.2%	25.2%

Obese Americans	Men	Women
Whites	20.8%	23.2%
Blacks	21.3%	38.2%
Hispanics	24.8%	36.1%

*Includes persons classified as *obese,* as well as *overweight*

Source: *2002 Heart and Stroke Statistical Update*, American Heart Association

Bringing your weight to your ideal level reverses the unfavorable effects of obesity, lessening your risk of high blood pressure, heart attack, stroke, and death. What could be a more convincing set of reasons to become slim and trim?

Neither doctor nor patient should be fooled into this type of rationalization: "When you lose your excessive weight, your blood pressure will be all right." Unfortunately, we don't know positively that the patient will reach the target weight, or how long it will take to get there. And we can't be sure that weight control will produce normal blood pressure.

Treating high blood pressure with medication is easy and inexpensive. *CCWD!* discusses this matter in more detail. An important point is that your starting drug should be either a diuretic or a beta-blocker. Both have been around for decades and, as generic drugs, are inexpensive. A diuretic reduces the blood volume, which reduces blood pressure. A beta-blocker neutralizes the effect of adrenaline-like substances that the body produces, lowering both blood pressure and heart rate. The doctor will decide which agent to use first and when, if ever, to add the second drug. Let's hope he has not been lured by the siren song of pharmaceutical companies to use other, more expensive agents for blood pressure control instead of those I have just mentioned.

Type 2 diabetes (formerly called adult-onset diabetes) is increasing rapidly, due to the obesity epidemic. If you inherited a tendency to diabetes, there is only one way to delay its development or prevent it from ever occurring: *weight control.* Having diabetes makes your risk of heart attack as great as in a person who has already had one or more previous heart attacks! If you should ever develop diabetes, weight control is an important part of its treatment. Why not control weight now and avoid diabetes entirely?

Keep from wearing out your weight-bearing joints. Carrying excessive weight for years puts a strain on your weight-bearing joints (hips and knees) with every step. The layer of cartilage that lines the joint becomes thinner and thinner until it may be worn away completely, resulting in a "bone on bone" situation. All of this causes painful weight-bearing. Doctors now call this *degenerative joint disease* (DJD) because the joint lining degenerates (wears away). Decades ago DJD was called *osteoarthritis*, a term that always made me want to say, "Make up your mind!" because *osteo-* refers to bone, while *arthritis* means inflammation of a joint. In truth, there is little or no actual *inflammation* in this situation, just wearing away of the cartilage.

Thus to me seemed odd that the group called *nonsteroidal anti-inflammatory drugs* (sometimes abbreviated to "NSAIDs,") were touted for use in DJD. The first of these was ibuprofen (Motrin), followed by a series of others that included naproxen (Aleve). When prolonged use of NSAIDs tended to cause stomach ulcers, which sometimes bled, the drug industry developed another generation of similar anti-inflammatory agents, even more expensive and currently frantically competing (Celebrex vs. Vioxx) for your prescription drug dollars by advertising to the public. Unfortunately, even these drugs have at times been associated with stomach ulceration and bleeding, although not as often as the earlier drugs.

To me, it has never made much sense to use an anti-inflammatory drug for a disorder with such a small inflammatory component. The truth is that all NSAIDs are quite effective *pain relievers*. It is this property that makes them useful. Nothing wrong with that, but why not prevent DJD in the first place? You can do that by reaching and maintaining your ideal weight.

Don't count on weight reduction to control your cholesterol. *Cholesterol Control Without Diet! The Niacin Solution* explains this fully. If diet reduces cholesterol at all, it usually does so only during periods of weight reduction. When the weight levels off, whether at the target level or only partway there, the cholesterol factory builds the cholesterol level back to where it was. A large community study showed that the American Heart Association (AHA) Step One diet (recommended for everyone) reduced cholesterol by a trivial amount. Even the stricter Step Two Diet (recommended for high-risk individuals) only lowered cholesterol by 5%, not enough to make much difference. Furthermore, *it reduced the good (HDL) cholesterol* just as much as it reduced bad (LDL) cholesterol, an unfavorable situation.

An abnormal cholesterol pattern accompanies obesity in many persons. Diet is the *only* way to control *weight*, but to bring *good and bad cholesterol* to desirable levels and keep them there, one must *change the body factory*. Medication is the best way to accomplish this change. Niacin is the best medication. It requires knowledgeable medical supervision. Both the patient and the doctor need to read *CCWD!* and use its information.

Do You Have What It Takes to Lose All of Your Excessive Weight?

Yes, you do. You have a brain and the ability to learn the principles I teach you. These include strategies that will help you to form a new set of eating habits to replace the unsuitable habits that caused your excessive weight.

When people say, "I don't have any willpower," they are wrong. You *do* have the willpower; you must just choose to *use it every time* you make one choice or another that will determine whether you succeed or fail. If you do this, you *will* succeed.

Be tough. Say to yourself several times each day (every time you must decide between a good choice or a bad one), "I am too fat! Do I want to reach my ideal weight? *Yes, I do!*

Let's understand a basic fact for any weight reduction program. *Body weight behaves just like your bank balance.* It increases when you deposit more than you withdraw but decreases when you take out more than you deposit. When you eat fewer calories every day than your body burns as fuel, the body will burn fat to make up the deficit. You will become thinner.

Don't "go on a diet." I dislike the expression "going on a diet" because it sounds like an enforced, abnormal program—like a prison term—with a beginning and an end, presumably when the dieter reaches her weight goal. Actually, if she returns to her previous eating habits, she will regain the lost weight. Many people refer to this variation, often with wide weight swings, as the "yo-yo" effect. The reason for this analogy is obvious, as is the depressing connotation of this all-too-common phenomenon. For this reason, fad diets that come and go have no lasting effect. They do not offer a long-term way of life.

To lose weight and keep it off, you must trade old, unsuitable eating habits for a new set of habits. You will design your own program. After I teach you the basic principles, *you* must devise the plan that works for you. You must be tough enough to keep using your plan until you reach your ideal weight. Then finally, you must modify your weight-*losing* program to become your long-term weight-*maintaining* regimen.

Did I say "long-term?" The correct term for that final stage, *maintaining* your best weight once you have reached it, should really be *lifelong*. Right! Now let's get there and stay there!

What Is My Ideal Weight? Am I Overweight or Obese?

How should you determine whether you have too much fat and how much above your ideal weight you are? Over the years there have been various rules for ideal or excessive weight. I have always liked one that says if you were not overweight at ages 20-22, *that should be your ideal weight for life.*

For many years we used the Metropolitan Life Insurance Company's tables of "ideal" weights for each height. There were different tables for men and women, each tallied according to small, medium, and large frames. The trouble is that the tables must have represented the average of the general public, which even then was too fat. The weights were too high to be of real value in setting proper goals.

My office booklet mentioned the "pinch and poke" system. It encouraged patients to pinch and poke the flesh around the abdomen to see how much fat they could find. The saying was that "If you can pinch more than an inch, it's too much." This tells you, "I am too fat" but doesn't tell you how much or what your goal should be. Try it anyway.

The experts, meeting to express concern about the obesity epidemic and suggest remedies, have endorsed a system that is more quantitative and helps to set your goals. It's called the Body Mass Index (BMI) and has actually been used to evaluate weight since the 1980's.

Here's how it works. Because it started in countries that express weight in kilograms and height in meters, it called for dividing the weight in kilograms by the square of the height in meters. **Table 2**, converted to US measures (pounds and inches), lets you find your BMI.

To do so, find your height in inches in the left column. Then locate the weight closest to yours in the line across the top of the page. This will let you locate your BMI. Overweight has been

Table 2

Adult Body Mass Index (BMI)

Height	Weight (pounds)						
	120	130	140	150	160	170	180
4' 6"	29	31	34	36	39	41	44
4' 8"	27	29	31	34	36	38	40
4' 10"	25	27	29	31	34	36	38
5' 0"	23	25	27	29	31	33	35
5' 2"	22	24	26	27	29	31	33
5' 4"	21	22	24	26	28	29	31
5' 6"	19	21	23	24	26	27	29
5' 8"	18	20	21	23	24	26	27
5' 10"	17	19	20	21	23	24	26
6' 0"	16	18	19	20	22	23	24
6' 2"	15	17	18	19	21	22	23
6' 4"	15	16	17	18	20	21	22
6' 6"	14	15	16	17	19	20	21
6' 8"	13	14	15	17	18	19	20

HEALTHY WEIGHT	OVERWEIGHT	OBESE
BMI 19-24	BMI 25-29	BMI 30+

(Table 2 is continued on next page)

Table 2 (continued)

Adult Body Mass Index (BMI)

Weight (pounds)

Height	190	200	210	220	230	240	250
4' 6"	46	48	51	53	56	58	60
4' 8"	43	45	47	49	52	54	56
4' 10"	40	42	44	46	48	50	52
5' 0"	37	39	41	43	45	47	49
5' 2"	35	37	38	40	42	44	46
5' 4"	33	34	36	38	40	41	43
5' 6"	31	32	34	36	37	39	40
5' 8"	29	30	32	34	35	37	38
5' 10"	27	29	30	32	33	35	36
6' 0"	26	27	28	30	31	33	34
6' 2"	24	26	27	28	30	31	32
6' 4"	23	24	26	27	28	29	30
6' 6"	22	23	24	25	27	28	29
6' 8"	21	22	23	24	25	26	29

HEALTHY WEIGHT	OVERWEIGHT	OBESE
BMI 19-24	BMI 25-29	BMI 30+

Source: *The Surgeon General's Call to Action to Prevent and Decrease Overweight and Obesity 2001* (US Department of Health and Human Services)

defined as a **BMI of 25 to 29.9**, Obesity is an excess of total body fat that results in a **BMI of 30 or more**.

Measuring Your Height and Weight Accurately. You need to check height only once, at the outset of your program, so be sure you do it correctly. Back up against a wall (in bare feet or thin socks) and have some one measure your height to the nearest half inch. You may be surprised to learn that you are not quite as tall as you thought you were. The older we get, the more likely this is to be so. As we grow older, the pads between the vertebrae lose their elasticity and become thinner. If each pad (*intervertebral disk*, if you are an anatomy buff or just like big words) thins out by only 1/30 of an inch, you lose an inch in height. In persons with osteoporosis, a compression fracture can crunch down the body of a vertebra by a greater amount, sometimes half an inch or more. And some persons have multiple compression fractures. So let's start with an accurately measured height.

To check your starting weight and follow your progress, be sure you have a good bathroom scale. It doesn't have to be the most expensive, but it should be easy to stand on and easy to read. Make sure your scale is well balanced on a firm surface (tile or wood, not carpet) and facing the same direction each time you weigh in for the record. You will be using the scale frequently to follow your progress.

Measuring your waistline. There's one more thing you need to measure: *your waist circumference*. The presence of excessive fat in the abdomen, out of proportion to total body fat, is an independent predictor of heart attack risk. Thus fat located in the abdominal region (sometimes referred to as "apple shape") is associated with greater health risk than that in peripheral regions, mainly the buttocks and thighs ("pear shape"). Measure waist circumference at the upper edge of the pelvis, a bone that is usually not difficult to feel, even in very obese persons. If you are in the lower part of the overweight range but have a pot belly, you need to check your waist measurement before treatment and follow it as you proceed with your reduction program.

The waist measurements that are associated with excess risk of heart disease are **more than 40 inches for men, more than 35 inches for women.**

Who is overweight and who is obese? Overweight has been defined as a **BMI of 25 to 29.9, obesity** as a **BMI of 30 or more.** There are a few limitations to this use of BMI. For example, it overestimates body fat in persons who are very muscular and can underestimate body fat in persons who have lost muscle mass (the elderly, or persons with enforced inactivity after surgery or prolonged illness). Don't be surprised that current BMI standards would classify both Sammy Sosa and Arnold Schwartzenegger as obese, Michael Jordan and Brad Pitt as overweight. But all that doesn't matter for most of us who are not trained athletes or body-builders. So learn and accept what your BMI is now; then let's work to lower it.

If you bring your BMI to less than 25, you will no longer be classified as overweight. At this point you must decide how far below this you want your body weight to be, to achieve all your goals, including looking as slim and trim as you would like.

How will you follow your progress? Weigh *several days in a row* before starting your program, to decide what is the most suitable weight to list as your starting point. Weight does vary a pound or two from day to day. If you were to weigh daily after beginning your program, you will notice this up-and-down bobble, which has no meaning and may distract you. Always weigh first thing in the morning, your lowest and most accurate weight of the day. There's no real need to weigh daily, but many people do this.

Weigh once a week for the record. Select one day of the week and make it your day to weigh in. Start your progress diary with your starting weight and BMI. You may also want to record the weight that will give you a BMI of 25 or less, considering this your goal. When you get there, you may decide to change your target weight to a lower level, to achieve the shape you desire. But getting the BMI to less than 25 is a milestone; if you are obese, getting it to below 30 is an important first step.

If you are doing everything properly, don't worry if you don't see as much loss as expected, especially at first. Sometimes fluid retention will temporarily mask the loss of fat, but the full amount of fat lost will be evident as soon as this extra fluid leaves the body—probably in the next week. For this reason, you may lose "inches before pounds." Stick to your program and the pounds will disappear.

How Can You Reach and Maintain Your Ideal Weight?

We have come this far without talking about calories, except in passing. Now we have to find out what calories are, where they abound, and how you can keep your daily intake of food energy, measured in calories, low enough to lose weight consistently.

What are calories? A calorie is a unit of energy used to express both the fuel value of foods and the amount of fuel energy the body uses. If you eat fewer calories than the body cells burn, weight loss results. Remember your bank balance? Many persons gradually gain weight over the years by becoming less active while continuing to eat amounts and types of food that maintained a stable weight in earlier, more active years. Often they combine this reduction in activity with subtle (or not so subtle) increases in habitual food intake. This helps to accumulate weight faster and keep it longer.

The *only* measure that accomplishes weight reduction is *calorie control.* Trust me: Exercise is a *fitness* maneuver but not really a *weight-losing* maneuver. Why do I say that? Now don't get me wrong. I *do* recommend regular physical activity; daily is best. But let's not fool ourselves about how many calories we are burning and think that exercise makes a great difference.

When I go to my workout place, if I walk on the treadmill for 30 minutes at 3.5 miles per hour and a 2% grade, *I burn just over 100 calories!* Not very much, is it? But I hate the treadmill, so for cardiovascular and leg exercise I usually ride the LifeCycle instead. If I ride 5 miles at about 70 revolutions per minute, which takes about 14 minutes, *I burn only 74 calories!* I rest my case.

So don't think of exercise as contributing significantly to your weight reduction program. If you do, there's a danger that you may say to yourself, "I've been so good with exercise that it doesn't matter if I have that cookie"—(or piece of pie, or whatever). *It does matter!* This kind of poorly informed rationalization can ruin a program.

Despite all this, exercise that makes the heart beat faster and the breathing rate increase ("cardiovascular exercise") *is* important for fitness. It contributes *a little* to the balance of calories eaten and used. *Mainly, it is symbolic of your dedication to the entire program.* You are determined to lose your weight and improve your fitness at the same time. Exercise *does* lessen the risk of cardiovascular disease to some extent. Walking 30 minutes a day, 5-7 days a week (7 is best, of course) should be part of your life. *Get tough and do it.* Once you build it into your daily schedule, continuing is easy. You notice that you feel better, stronger, more energetic. That's what fitness is. Never mind that it doesn't help a lot in weight loss. It helps a little, and these other rewards make it worthwhile. In the fall of 2002, an advisory committee from the Institute of Medicine actually advocated increasing daily exercise for both adults and children to *one hour a day*. More of this later.

Now back to foods and calories. The major food classes are *proteins, carbohydrates, and fats.* To plan your weight reduction program, you need to know their relative values in calories.

Let's compare the fuel value of *one gram* (1/30 ounce) of each:

Protein	4 calories
Carbohydrate	4 calories
Fat	9 calories

As you see, any fat you eat contains many more calories (225% as many, in fact) as the same weight of protein or carbohydrate. This explains why cutting fat to a minimum is a key part of any weight reduction program.

Your body has plenty of stored fat which, unfortunately, also has this high fuel value, 9 calories per gram. To burn much of this high-calorie fuel requires a deficit of many calories over a considerable period of time. For this reason, weight reduction usually proceeds slowly, seldom more than 1 to 1.5 pounds a week.

Any faster weight loss involves a certain amount of "fake" loss because semi-starvation causes loss of fluid and even loss of muscle. These fake losses return when you resume adequate eating. So please resist the urge to try fad diets or semi-starvation. If living mainly on grapefruit or on cabbage soup promoted real and healthful weight loss, the obesity epidemic would be history—and it isn't.

Weight loss plans that promise greater losses in shorter times are all around us. Don't be fooled by centers that charge nominal amounts for weight reduction, "plus the cost of food." They may give some instruction but are basically food stores that provide low-calorie food at a premium price. Their defect is that they don't instill the necessary information to reach ideal weight and then maintain it for a lifetime. By providing all of your food they omit the most important feature—education to make your results last. Notice that their TV pitch, with before and after pictures, often bears the disclaimer, "Results not typical." Of course these food stores select their most striking successes (and most photogenic people) for their ads. But what about the others that don't fare as well? We never hear about them. And how many of those who do reach their weight goals fail to maintain that ideal weight?

The basic principle is: If [put in the name of the advertised product or system] were as effective as they say, everyone would know about it and nearly everyone would be using it. I won't waste much space (or your reading time) by listing and commenting on the seductive ads touting easy ways to lose a lot of weight. But here are a few samples, taken from newspapers, the Internet, or TV. Do these sound credible to you?

- "No dieting, no exercising! Would you like to lose weight while you sleep? Body fat loss, wrinkle reduction, energy level, muscle strength, sexual potency, emotional stability, memory [all improved]." This is an ad for a product said to release human growth hormone (HGH) and is complete with a list of old movie stars and aging world political leaders who had received injected HGH, according to Mike Wallace (CBS, *Sixty Minutes*).

- "Do you need to safely lose weight fast?" This ad is for a mixture of eight amino acids (the building blocks of protein) of vegetable origin, "in a perfect ratio....Only one calorie per dose!" The nutritional product is said to be the equivalent of eating 350 grams (11-12 ounces) of poultry, fish, or meat. It is illustrated with a picture of a woman in a two-piece bathing suit and a man in trunks, neither of them wearing an ounce of excess fat.

- "Lose 6-20 inches in one hour guaranteed." This headlines an ad for "our slenderizing mineral body wrap," called "safe, healthy, and hydrating." It is said to "reduce cellulite while it tightens and tones the skin." Of course, the "lose inches" gimmick is reached by adding the inches lost at many sites, but even so, 6 to 20 inches in an hour defies belief.

I promised not to waste your time, so no more of this nonsense. I trust you will resolve not to be taken in by unbelievable pitches. Whether the American public spends $58 billion or closer to $30 billion annually on weight-loss products and programs doesn't matter; both figures are ridiculous. What matters is the 98% failure rate. Don't be a part of it.

Who controls honesty in advertising? The Federal Trade Commission (FTC) does. In the fall of 2002 they reported that companies were using phony ads and misleading claims to dupe fat people into buying their products, despite increased FTC enforcement actions. Their report did not single out specific products, companies or ads. They did study about 300 ads in 2001. The FTC said that 55% of the weight-loss ads made claims that lack proof or likely were false, such as "I lost 46 pounds in 30 days!" My guess is that the 55% figure should be closer to 100%.

The wire service story said that FTC, when pressed for examples of deceptive ads, cited a list on the agency's web site of several dozen recent cases in which it was pursuing enforcement. These included products called "Fat Trapper" and "Exercise in a

Bottle," as well as abdominal machines that promised tight abdominal muscles ("washboard abs") through electrical stimulation.

FTC compared ads in specific publications in 1992 and in 2001. They found that in 1992 most ads (57%) were for lower-calorie meal replacements; by 2001, two-thirds of ads were for dietary supplements that claimed that diet and exercise were completely unnecessary. Some ads claimed weight losses of 8 to 10 pounds a week, far more than experts agree is realistic.

Now let's talk about the only approach that *does* work. To be successful, a program for lasting weight reduction must be practical as a way of life, to be used daily as long as necessary to lose the desired amount of weight. You must plan it carefully. An average loss of *4 to 5 pounds a month* is the best that most people can achieve. Using the BMI table, find out how many pounds you must lose to reach a "healthy" weight (BMI of less than 25). You can then divide this projected weight loss by 4 or 5 for a rough estimate of how many months it will take to lose your excess weight—if you do well.

Are carbohydrate and protein really equal? Although protein and carbohydrate are equal in caloric content, 4 calories per gram, they are handled differently by the body. Protein is needed to replace muscle cells and thus protect against having body muscle depleted by a marked calorie deficit, as mentioned before. Carbohydrate is burned rapidly to meet energy needs, and some is stored in the liver, to be released if the blood sugar falls too low. Any excess is stored as fat.

The body uses or stores carbohydrate (starches and sugars) fairly rapidly, with the blood sugar returning to fasting levels within two hours after a meal, except in diabetics. Sugars are absorbed and raise the blood sugar more rapidly than starches, which have to be converted into sugars by digestive enzymes before being absorbed. Protein (meat, poultry, fish, eggs) is used more slowly over several hours, which prevents early return of hunger or appetite. **Figure 1** illustrates these differences in time of utilization and satisfaction of hunger and appetite.

Which of these breakfasts would be more likely to keep you from becoming hungry in mid-morning?
(A) Orange juice, cereal with sugar and milk, toast, jelly, coffee; or
(B) orange juice, one or two eggs, lean breakfast meat, toast, coffee?

If you aren't sure, you might want to try each breakfast and see. Or you may know from experience that the protein breakfast (B) will "stay with you" longer, while the carbohydrate breakfast (A) will probably leave you hungry by mid-morning. The carbohydrate eater feels hungry, looks at her watch, and finds that it is only 10:30. What to do? Too often this leads to a mid-morning

Figure 1

Satisfaction from Consuming Sugar, Starch, or Protein

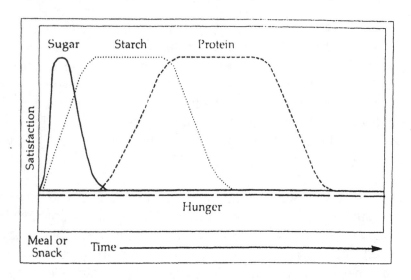

Source: *Child of Mine: Feeding with Love and Good Sense,*
by Ellyn Satter, RD, MS (Nutrition), MS (Social Work).
Used with permission.

snack, maybe a sweet roll or Danish with coffee (sugar? cream?), or a calorie-containing beverage such as a non-diet soda. When the protein eater feels hungry, her watch says that it is noon and time to go to lunch. That's why protein is an important part of breakfast—and of all meals, for that matter.

The next step: designing your own program. I want you to design your own set of eating habits (or dietary program, but not "diet," please). Are you ready to get tough with excess fat? Here are some rules to start with:

- *No butter, margarine, or things made with shortening* (cakes, pies, cookies). Eat bread, toast, or rolls *without butter or margarine*, enjoying the flavor of the baked goods. Avoid croissants, which contain lots of butter. If you *must* spread something on your bread or roll, use the thinnest possible layer of jam or jelly, which is much lower in calories than butter or margarine. Try the excellent low-calorie jams made by Smucker's or Knott's Berry Farm.

- Cut all visible fat from meat and remove skin from poultry. Broil meats (as on a grill), so the fat will liquefy and drip away.

- *There is no place for alcohol in a weight reduction program.* Yes, you read that correctly. ***There is no place for alcohol in a weight reduction program.*** Be tough! Here are three reasons to avoid alcohol:

    (1)   It contains calories.
    (2)   It stimulates appetite.
    (3)   It reduces willpower.

Later we'll discuss this matter in more detail, including a possible compromise.

- *Don't skip breakfast.* That maneuver almost certainly dooms a program to failure.

- Choose protein (eggs, lean meat) for most meals, including breakfast.

- Choose starches in preference to sweets, as a general rule. Unless you are allergic, *drink milk.* To keep fat and calories low, use 1% milk. Skim milk and buttermilk (which contain no fat) are slightly lower in calories, but there's no need to go that far unless you don't mind the taste. Both 2% and 4% (the latter usually labeled just "homogenized milk") have too much fat and too many calories for your program.

•   Eat fruits and vegetables. Dietitians recommend four to five servings a day, which isn't difficult to achieve. In general, fruits and vegetables are low in calories, are filling, and contain important nutrients (vitamins and fiber).

•   Use fruits as desserts and as a planned afternoon snack. Use vegetables that have practically no calories for nibbles or snacks rather than calorie-rich candies or the like.

•   Salads often can be an entire meal, keeping calories low and satisfying part of your daily goal for fruits and vegetables. But watch salad dressings carefully. Unless specifically labeled "low-calorie" dressings, they are often high in calories, more than all the rest of the meal together. Read the labels! Vinegar contains no calories, and many delicious types are available.

•   Drink enough water to satisfy thirst. Some recommend drinking water frequently through the day to keep feeling full instead of hungry. If it works for you, fine. Happily, that old edict of eight to ten glasses of water every day has finally been abandoned. Such an excess of water can, in fact, be harmful in some people, reducing their blood sodium levels.

Special strategies for your weight reduction program. Before getting into calorie mathematics, let me strongly advise several strategies that will reduce your food intake. Regardless of your food choices, these maneuvers will put you on the road to effective weight reduction. Start immediately.

♦   *Buy small!*—not the largest banana, apple, melon, other.

♦   Cook smaller amounts of food. Same reasoning.

♦   No nibbling while cooking.

♦   *Use smaller plates*. What you serve then seems like more food. You soon become used to the smaller amounts. Fill any gaps with low-calorie vegetables.

♦   Serve plates at the stove. *Serve only 2/3 of the amounts you formerly ate. For some foods, you may be able to reduce to half-*

portions right away. Eventually try to reduce portions to less than two-thirds of your old eating habits.

♦　　　No food on the table to invite second helpings.

♦　　　No second helpings.

♦　　　*Take smaller bites.*

♦　　　*Do not prepare the next bite,* cutting or putting onto your fork, *until after you have chewed and swallowed the current one.* This takes some practice, but you can do it. Making this a habit will help you to lose weight.

♦　　　*Put your silverware down between bites.* This will make you take longer to eat, which is part of our strategy. Again, this takes practice. It is important.

♦　　　Stop eating when you feel *satisfied, not stuffed.* Eating rapidly, to the point of feeling stuffed, is a contributing cause of obesity.

♦　　　Leave some food on your plate. The old-fashioned "clean your plate" ethic has contributed to the obesity epidemic. Maybe your parents, like mine, used the "clean your plate" plan, sometimes adding, "If you eat a good dinner, you may have dessert." Did they?

♦　　　Along with taking longer to eat, aim for a relaxed atmosphere. Maybe not candlelight (although what's wrong with that?), but music is better than TV news, a nonsensical sitcom, or other distraction. And be sure to avoid arguments or other unpleasantness. Families should eat together and talk to each other.

♦　　　No nibbling while cleaning up the dishes. Either refrigerate leftovers or grind them. Your garbage disposer was made to handle those leftover nibbles; to your body they represent extra, uncounted calories.

♦　　　No candy dishes or similar temptations like snack machines, at home or at work. Learn to say "no" to yourself each time you see such a temptation. Tell yourself, "I am too fat, and I am simply not going to do it!" Every time you pass up such a temptation, you gain more respect for your willpower and determination. This self-esteem makes it even easier to say "no" the next time.

♦   *No samples at the grocery*, no matter how good they look or how hungry you are. (Why are you shopping when hungry anyhow?) If you try one of those tempting samples, you will forget you had it and will fail to count the calories. A basic principle for weight loss is to *never eat an unplanned or uncounted calorie.*

♦   Don't eat in the car. You tend to eat more and faster, than in other settings. If you are the driver, surveys show that eating in the car is just as risky as using a cell phone. *Don't do it.* For others, it eliminates the delaying strategies of not preparing the next bite and of putting silverware down between bites.

By using these strategies effectively and daily, you will automatically begin to lose weight, even if you were to continue to eat the same foods you have eaten until now. Now let's think about food selections that can make even a greater difference in your fuel intake This is the official beginning of your journey to reach your ideal weight and maintain it.

How to Control Your Intake of Calories

Here's where you have to use your brain and a little math—which, fortunately, is not complicated. You don't need to write down everything you eat and calculate the calories, although some find this helpful, at least at first. Here's a good rule: *Know at least the approximate caloric content of everything you eat.* Everything!

This may sound difficult, but it isn't. Many foods have the calorie content printed on their labels. To tell how calorie-rich a food is, what's the first thing you look at on the label? Calories? No. Calories from fat? No. It is the *serving size*. Then look at the calories, and you know how much food equals that number.

If you look at the calories first, here's how you can be fooled. I just looked at the labels of two salad dressings, a Thousand Island and a Ranch dressing. The labels showed 120 and 130 calories per serving, respectively. But what about the serving size? In each case, "2 tblsp." Who puts only two tablespoonfuls of dressing on his salad? That's an ounce, 30 cc, or 2/3 of a shot glass. Even fat-free California French dressing contains 45 calories in 2 tblsp. A good plan would be to use a favorite vinegar, chosen from many on the grocer's shelves, with no calories. By such calorie-awareness, you will put together your calorie-saving program.

You definitely should have a good book of caloric values. Although there are little calorie booklets at the grocery checkout counter, I urge you just once to spend a small amount for a complete guide that will help you in many ways. I recommend for you the book I recently bought, *The Doctor's Pocket Calorie Fat & Carbohydrate Counter,* by Allan Borushek. It is a colorful 4 x 6 paperback book bearing a 2002 copyright and containing a wealth of calorie information. You'll find it easy to look up the caloric content of *every food you eat*—which is exactly what you need to do to succeed. There are also brief guides to calcium and sodium, which you don't need for weight control but about which I will comment before we are finished. Perhaps its best feature, which puts it ahead of other books in this field, is its *very* complete listing of fast-food chains and restaurants—101 of them! Would you have guessed that there were that many?

This little book is so complete that at first glance it may appear too formidable. It's not. Buy it and use it. Do you think you will have trouble remembering how many calories are in the foods you eat? Let me give you some words of reassurance about that.

Let's face this fact: Calorie designations are approximate, not exact. They're pretty good. Those published in a guide this good are very useful, and that's all that matters. Bear in mind that a "medium banana" means different things to different people. Same for other fruits and many other things that come in different sizes. (That's why we taught you to "buy small." It saves more calories.)

Obviously it matters more that you learn the calories in the foods you eat most often, many of them every day—or avoid every day, as in the case of butter, margarines, and other shortenings. Both for your own benefit and to help friends and relatives, I encourage you to take a lined sheet of paper and make a list of the caloric contents of foods you eat often. Then you won't have to keep looking them up until they are imprinted in your mind. Make a separate list of foods that are high in calories and which, therefore, you have decided to avoid entirely. From time to time you may want to share some of this information with others who are heading toward ideal weight. It will also serve to remind you why you put foods onto this list.

I will do part of the work for you by giving you some of the information that you will find useful. You will do the rest for yourself.

How many calories per day? Rather than prescribing a daily level of calories, I advise that you *substantially reduce your intake of calories below the level that has been holding your weight steady.* When I practiced in a clinic group, dietitians converted my dietary prescriptions into a practical program for each patient. I usually prescribed *1000 calories a day* for the housewife or a business woman of average height or less, with little exercise apart from work. For taller or more active women and for most business men, I prescribed *1200 calories a day.* For tall men or physical laborers, *1400-1500 calories a day* usually works.

As you plan your program, these figures can be a general guide to keep in mind as you look at the caloric values of foods. For practical purposes, most people can think of *1200 calories a day* as an estimated goal. It helps you to put a Big Mac (590*) and large fries (540*) into perspective, doesn't it? More about fast foods later.

How to lose four to six pounds a month. If your weight has been stable recently, your caloric intake and expenditure have, over a period of time, been equal. The intelligent changes in eating habits that you have already begun to devise will reduce your intake by hundreds of calories each day while you still have plenty to eat. If you *consistently* reduce your previous habits by an average of *500 calories each day* (not hard to do), in a week you will have a net deficit of 3500 calories. *Each time you accumulate a net deficit of 3500 calories, you lose one pound.* If you can trim your daily intake by an average of *700 calories a day* (which for some means only giving up alcohol, desserts, or snacks), you will reach a net deficit of 3500 calories in only five days.

By consistently making reductions of 3500 calories each five to seven days, you can lose four to six pounds a month for as long as necessary to reach your goal. Most people can't trim weight any faster than this, although some do if the previous intake has been very high and they do a good job of cutting back. Just getting rid of alcohol and bedtime snacks can do this for some people. But across-the-board calorie reductions are even better. *Be tough!*

*Yes, numbers in parentheses show the caloric content of each item

Now let's talk about *how* to reduce calories; first general principles, then details.

Reducing your intake of fats. Remember the first lesson in calories: fat contains 225% as many calories as the same weight of protein or carbohydrate. Therefore, you will achieve major savings in calories by reducing your fat intake to a low level. How can you accomplish this? If we have already mentioned some items, please bear with me. I am including them now so this list will be complete.

1.   Trim all visible fat from meat. Buy meat that looks lean instead of being heavily marbled with fat. (But that doesn't matter much if you broil the meat on your grill, so the fat melts and drips off instead of going into your body.)

2.   Don't buy already-ground hamburger from your grocer's display. Even the package labeled "our leanest" contains a fair amount of visible fat, doesn't it? Instead, choose a lean cut of round steak or chuck. Ask the butcher to trim all of the visible fat, then grind the beef for you. This gives you fat-free ground meat for your hamburgers or casseroles.

3.   Avoid bacon and sausage, both of which contain entirely too much fat. As your breakfast meats, use part of a lean ham slice or a small breakfast steak. Canadian bacon costs more than fatty bacon strips but is a better buy if you consider lean protein content. It doesn't take a very large portion of any of these lean meats, eaten with an egg, to satisfy hunger and provide ample protein.

4.   Avoid processed lunch meats. They all contain too much fat.

5.   Don't fry or deep-fry. Broil meats; bake potatoes. No french-fries.

6.   Keep the fat content of your milk as low as you find practical. Never use more than 2% milk. And 1% tastes just as good. Skim milk and buttermilk contain no fat. You Avoid cookies, cakes, pies, other baked goods—mainly because they contain butter or shortening but also because of carbohydrate calories.

7.   Avoid nuts, high in calories because of their high content of fatty oils.

8.   Try to eliminate table spreads (butter, margarine) entirely. This can save thousands of calories over time, especially if you have previously used them heavily. Ordinary butter has about 100 calories per pat (1 tblsp.), light or whipped butter about 70 calories per tblsp. If you have used several pats a day, you can save hundreds of calories every day by avoiding them entirely. Instead of putting butter or sour cream on baked potatoes, season the potatoes with pepper, a little salt, or experiment with other spices. Instead of butter on vegetables, try other seasonings: vinegar, lemon juice, herbs, spices.

9.   Use the lowest-calorie salad dressing you can find, or make your own from readily available recipes. (Before we're through, we'll give you one in this booklet.) Vinegars taste good and contain no calories.

Spreading your food intake through the day. As you plan your weight control program, your food intake should be divided fairly equally among three or more meals. Do not skip breakfast or skimp on protein at either breakfast or lunch. Some persons try to lose weight by skipping breakfast, skimping on lunch, and eating practically all their day's calories at supper. And, of course, they overeat, because by then they are ravenous. They rationalize: "I've been so good all day that it doesn't matter if I eat more for supper." But it does.

If you feed the same total calories for the day to two groups of laboratory animals but allow one group to nibble all day, while the other group gets their feeding all at one time, the one-meal group tends to gain weight more than the daylong nibblers. It is unusual for a person who eats only one meal a day to lose weight effectively.

Emphasizing protein. Be sure your meals are built around adequate amounts of protein (lean meat, poultry, fish, eggs, or low-calorie cheese). We have already discussed breakfast protein (lean meat, eggs). In planning the protein foundation of other meals, remember that even good protein sources contain calories. Lean beef has about 60 calories per ounce, so three ounces contains 180 calories and can be quite satisfying. However, if you eat six or eight ounces, you take in 360 to 480 calories, about a third of your daily target amount. Cottage cheese, at 30 calories per ounce (one rounded tablespoon) is fine, but if you eat a lot of it, the calories begin to add up. Even so, it is a lot lower than cheddar, American, or Swiss cheeses, all at 100 to 110 calories per ounce.

Now is as good a time as any to be sure you aren't laboring under the delusion that it's wrong to eat eggs or red meat. True, the greatest source of actual cholesterol in our diets is egg yolk. But here's what you need to know: The body manufactures most of its cholesterol, at least 80% of it. How much cholesterol you eat (as in eggs) really doesn't make any difference in your blood cholesterol. *CCWD!* cites a study in which healthy young men were divided into three groups; one group ate three eggs a week, another group seven eggs a week, and the third group fourteen eggs a week. At the end of the five-month study, *all three groups had the same levels of total cholesterol and of LDL ("bad") cholesterol.* There are numerous other studies showing how little eggs matter. So go ahead; *eat eggs and enjoy them.* There is no reason even to think of spending money on products consisting of egg whites alone. Eggs are an important source of protein and can be served in so many ways that they should be a part of your dietary program, at any time of day, perhaps on a daily basis. *Enjoy eggs!*

Most people don't know that *lean red meat is interchangeable with chicken on AHA diets*. It is. I don't know how the superstition that red meats are bad for you got started, but it is not true. Enjoy lean red meats!

Adding carbohydrate. Remember that carbohydrates are no higher in calories than protein, gram for gram, so it's not sinful to include them in limited amounts. Starches are better than sweets, however. Breads, dry or cooked cereals, rice, any pasta, crackers, potatoes, corn, or beans can all add variety to the program. (Beans add protein as well.) There's no need to eliminate bread if you omit the butter and jelly, or to eliminate potatoes if you don't add gravy, butter, or sour cream.

Fruits and vegetables. Dietitians are unanimous in advising liberal use of fruits and vegetables for everyone, whether seeking weight reduction or not. It is easy to achieve their recommended "at least 4 to 5 servings of fruits and vegetables daily."

Tables 3 and 4 show the caloric values of many fruits and vegetables. Notice that many fruits and (particularly) vegetables

Table 3
Caloric Values of Fruits

Type of Fruit	Calories
Apple, fresh, medium	90
Apricot, canned, in water	35
in juice, halves w/skin, 1cup	120
dried, 8 halves	65
Avocado, 1 fruit, 6 oz	300
Banana, 1 medium, 3 per pound	80
Blackberry, fresh, 1 cup	75
Blueberry, fresh, 1 cup	80
Boysenberry, canned, light syrup, 1 cup	120
Cantaloupe, ¼ medium (or cubed, 1 cup)	55

Table 3 (continued)

Type of Fruit	Calories
Cherry, fresh, sweet, 8 (2 oz)	40
Royal Anne, pitted, heavy syrup, ½ cup	110
Grapefruit, white or pink, ½ large	40
Mulberry, raw, 20 berries, 1 oz	15
Orange, 3", 7 oz	70
Orange juice, 8 oz	110
Peach, fresh, large, 6 oz	55
canned, in juice, 1 cup	100
Pear, fresh, 1 medium, 6 oz	90
canned, halves, in juice, ½ cup	60
Pineapple, fresh, diced, 1 cup	80
canned, chunks, in juice, ½ cup	70
Plum, fresh, 2 medium	90
canned, in juice or light syrup, 3 plums w/liquid	85
Prune, dried, pitted, 4 medium, 1 oz	70
canned, in syrup, 4 prunes	120
Raspberry, fresh, 1 cup	60
Strawberry, halves, 1 cup	45
Tangerine, fresh, raw, 1 medium, 4 oz	50
sections, canned, light syrup, ½ cup	80
Watermelon, fresh: 1" slice, 10" diameter	70
balls or diced, 1 cup	50

Table 4
Caloric Values of Vegetables

Type of Vegetable	Calories
Acorn squash, raw, ½ medium, 10 oz	85
Artichoke, raw, 1 medium, 4.5 oz	65
Asparagus, fresh, 4 spears	15
canned, ½ cup	20
frozen, 1 cup	50
Beets, boiled, drained, sliced, ½ cup	25
Broccoli, boiled, 1 medium stalk, 5 oz	40
Butternut squash, baked, cubed, 1 cup	80

Table 4 (continued)

Type of Vegetable	Calories
Cabbage, fresh, shredded, ½ cup	8
Cabbage, red, fresh, shredded, ½ cup	10
Carrot, fresh, 7" x 1 ¼" diameter	33
canned, ½ cup	35
Cauliflower, 1/2 medium head, 15 oz	100
Celery, raw, strips, 1 cup	10
Corn, 1 ear, 5-6"	80
½ cup	65
Cucumber, peeled, sliced, 1 cup	5
Green beans, canned, ½ cup	20
Lettuce, iceberg, 1 leaf	3
romaine, 6 leaves	20
Mushroom, canned/jars, ½ cup	20
Peas, green, canned, ½ cup	60
Pepper, sweet, green or red, sliced, 1 cup	25
Potato, unpeeled, baked, 7 oz	90
canned, 16 oz.	200
mashed, w/milk & butter, ½ cup	110
Rice, white, 1 cup, "Boiler Bag"	190
Spinach, raw, 3 oz	40
boiled, drained, 1 cup	50
canned, ½ cup	25
Sweet potato, baked in skin, 1 large	120
Mashed, ½ cup	170
Tomato, ripe, fresh: red, raw, 2 ½" diameter	35
red, raw, cherry tomato, 1 cup	30
red, stewed, 1 cup	60
sun-dried, 5-6 pc	22
Turnip, fresh or stored: cubed, 1 cup	30
Turnip greens, raw, chopped, 1 cup	15
boiled, drained, chopped, 1 cup	30
Watercress, fresh, chopped, 10 sprigs, 1 oz	4
Zucchini, boiled, drained, sliced, 1 cup	30

Source: Allan Borushek's *The Doctor's Pocket Calorie, Fat & Carbohydrate Counter*

are low in calories and can be mainstays of your program, both at meals and as snacks. One of your best strategies will be to reach for a low-calorie vegetable when you are hungry between meals or in the evening, rather than for the high-calorie snack food or candy that you may have chosen until now.

Filling, not fattening. Some foods have very few calories, often because they are high in fiber (in earlier decades called cellulose or "bulk"). My booklet always included a list of these so-called "zero-calorie" foods, which you may eat in unlimited quantities with meals or between meals. Here this information is in **Table 5** and **Table 6**. As I recall, Ellyn Satter (now a successful author) gave me this list and the accompanying few recipes to fill out my booklet when we were both at the Jackson Clinic (Madison, Wisconsin) in the late 1960's. They have remained in the booklet through numerous minor revisions since then, and I think readers will find them useful now. (To be precise, we should confess that the "zero-calorie" foods really have a few calories—but less than 10 per serving.) Use them to round out your meals or as snacks at any time you become hungry.

Table 5

FOODS VERY LOW IN CALORIES
(FOR USE IN WEIGHT REDUCTION PROGRAMS)

The following foods are very low in calories. You may eat them at any time, in any amount you desire. The vegetables listed may be eaten raw, canned, cooked, or frozen.

VEGETABLES	SOUPS, BEVERAGES, JUICES
Asparagus	Bouillon cubes
Bean sprouts	Coffee
Broccoli	Consomme
Cabbage	Lemonade*
Cauliflower	Lemon or lime juice
Cranberries*	Low calorie sodas
Celery	Tea
Celery cabbage	Tomato juice
Cucumber	V-8 juice
Endive (escarole)	* Artificially sweetened

Table 5 (continued)

Greens (mustard, kale, chard, etc.)
Green Pepper
Mushrooms
Okra
Onions, green
Peppers, pickled, hot

Pickles, dill
Pimiento
Parsley
Radishes
Rhubarb*
Sauerkraut

Spinach
String beans
Tomatoes
Water chestnuts
Watercress
Wax beans
* Artificially sweetened

DESSERTS AND JELLIES
Gelatin, unflavored
Jams and jellies, 1-2 calories

SEASONINGS

Garlic or onion juice
Herbs
Horseradish (not containing
   cream)
Mustard
Seasoning salts
Soy sauce
Spices
Vinegar
Worcestershire sauce

Table 6

LOW-CALORIE RECIPES

The following recipes show how low-calorie foods can be combined to make tasty dishes. Your ingenuity will suggest others.

TOMATO ASPIC SALAD

2 tblsp (2 envelopes) unflavored gelatin
1 tblsp onion juice
½ cup cold water
1 bay leaf
3 cups tomato juice

1/8 tsp cayenne pepper
½ cup chopped celery
1 dash black pepper
2 tblsp vinegar

Soften gelatin in cold water. Combine remaining ingredients. Heat to boiling, then simmer 10 minutes. Stir in softened gelatin until dissolved. Strain (if desired) and pour into I ½ quart mold. Chill until firm. This is delicious served with lean roast beef!

Table 6 (continued)

LOW-CALORIE RECIPES

MARINATED BEAN SALAD

1 can green beans, drained   1 can wax beans, drained
1 can water chestnuts, drained   1 can mushrooms, drained

  Chop together any desired amounts of celery, green onion, and green pepper. Mix all ingredients together with low-calorie Italian salad dressing. Add salt and pepper to taste. Refrigerate overnight. Serve.

BEAN-STUFFED TOMATOES (6 servings)

  Cook one 9-ounce package frozen Italian style green beans according to package directions. Drain thoroughly. Place in bowl with one 3-ounce can sliced mushrooms, drained. Add 1/3 cup low-calorie Italian dressing, ¼ cup sliced green onion, ¼ tsp salt, and a dash of pepper. Toss. Refrigerate for 2 hours, tossing occasionally.
  Meanwhile, cut a thin slice from the tops of 6 medium-size tomatoes and scoop out their centers, leaving shells about ¼ inch thick. Invert on paper towel to drain. Chill. At serving time, season shells with salt and fill with bean mixture.

WEIGHT-WATCHERS' SOUP

1 cup chopped celery, including leaves
1 bouillon cube (2nd cube may be used for added flavor)
1 cup chopped cabbage
¼ cup chopped onion   1 cup tomato juice
Salt and pepper to taste   2 cups water

  Simmer slowly for an hour. Refrigerate overnight. Heat to serve.

ZERO-CALORIE SALAD DRESSING

1 cup tomato juice
¼ cup lemon juice or vinegar (or both)
2 tblsp finely minced onion
Salt and pepper to taste

Cholesterol. Diet has so little to do with your cholesterol level that we might as well say that diet has nothing to do with cholesterol.. Sometimes weight reduction alone will reduce "bad" cholesterol. That's the good news. The bad news is that diet will usually control cholesterol only during periods of weight reduction, and you can't go on losing weight forever. When your weight levels off, whether at your target level or only partway there, your body factory makes the blood cholesterol level drift back to higher values. More bad news: diet, if it reduces cholesterol at all, usually reduces good cholesterol as much as bad cholesterol, an unfavorable situation.

Eat all the eggs you desire. Don't be fooled into buying any food because of a "low cholesterol" label. We have already mentioned that the amount of cholesterol you eat (of which egg yolks are the richest source) has little to do with your blood cholesterol level since the body manufactures most of its cholesterol. If you have a cholesterol problem—whether it is too much bad cholesterol, not enough good cholesterol, and/or triglycerides that are too high—you should read *Cholesterol Control Without Diet! The Niacin Solution.* That book teaches about cholesterol problems in easily understood words.

The long and the short of it is that cholesterol problems need to be treated by *changing the factory* that makes cholesterol in your body. This can best be done by medication, of which niacin has the longest safety record and was the first drug ever shown to reduce heart attacks, strokes, and deaths. It controls cholesterol inexpensively and without diet. What better news could there be, especially for American adults, burdened by high prescription costs and wary about deaths caused by the best-selling statin drugs?

Visit this web site to learn more about *Cholesterol Control Without Diet! The Niacin Solution* (and the book you are now reading), including ordering information:

w w w . c h o l e s t e r o l n o d i e t . c o m

Alcohol. As pointed out earlier, alcohol has no place in a weight-losing program, for three reasons:
(1) It contains calories.
(2) It stimulates appetite.
(3) It reduces willpower.
Is there a compromise that allows some alcohol? Let's discuss it.

All alcoholic drinks are relatively high in calories: about 146 in 12 ounces of beer, 100 in a "light" beer; 140 in a martini; about 120 in 1½ ounces of bourbon, scotch, rum, vodka, or tequila. Dry table wines have about 100 calories in a four-ounce glass. If we define a "drink" as 1½ ounces of hard liquor, 4 ounces of wine, or 12 ounces of beer, each has about the same alcohol content and about the same number of calories (120-150). Anyone who has been averaging more than two drinks a day, using this definition, should reduce his intake to two drinks a day or less. Consistent intake of more than that amount can damage liver, brain, or peripheral nerves. There is a test for early trouble in the liver but not the others. If you have customarily had two or more drinks a day, or even one, you can substantially reduce your total calories considerably by eliminating the alcohol.

During your *weight-losing* phase, I strongly recommend that you *select something with few or no calories* to replace alcoholic drinks. At social occasions when others are drinking, many persons sip beverages that resemble alcoholic drinks but are not: club soda, mineral water, one-calorie carbonated beverages, tomato juice, Bloody Mary mix. "Light" beers aren't that low in calories, so don't let that adjective fool you. If you want the taste of beer without the calories, a non-alcoholic beer is a better choice.

If you really can't bring yourself to eliminate alcohol entirely, sip a dry wine or have no more than one ounce of your favorite liquor with water or soda. But be prepared to have a slower weight loss than you would like, plus having to cut down more on other foods. Later, after reaching your desired weight, you will be able to include an alcoholic drink in your *weight-maintaining* program.

While we are talking about "just one ounce of liquor," let me caution you against *not knowing how much you are drinking*. I am talking about the drinker who does not measure with a shot glass as he makes a drink. How often have I asked a patient, "Do you measure the amount of liquor you put into your drink or just pour it, glug-glug-glug, from the bottle?" The usual answer was glug-glug-glug. So I have always advised *measuring each drink*. A "drink," as we define it, is 1½ ounces of liquor. If a person pours an unmeasured amount from the bottle into his glass, he does not know how much he is drinking, but you can bet it is more than 1½ ounces, especially after the first drink.

Remember that one reason to avoid alcohol on your weight-losing program is that it lowers willpower. You must *be tough* to limit to one drink a day, if that. But do it. If you are not tough enough to limit to one drink a day (or, even better, none), you probably will not succeed.

Examining your recent eating habits. To begin to decide where you can reduce calories, sit down and list on paper a day's intake that is typical of your recent eating pattern. Today's intake is easiest to recall. Be sure it is typical. Or fake a record, using foods from today and yesterday, just so you are honest with yourself. Don't forget to include snacks, soft drinks, and alcoholic beverages. *These are often the most opportune places to reduce calories significantly.* Then look up the caloric values for your typical day's eating, estimating portion sizes as best you can. Add up total calories and notice how they were distributed through the day. You will already be thinking of ways to redesign your program with substantially fewer calories.

How to get rid of the calories you'll never miss. For about eight years in the 1960's, the Pennwalt Corporation generously supplied copies of an excellent booklet, *Are You Really Serious About Losing Weight?* I used it with my office booklet until production costs forced them to discontinue their booklet. Although the company no longer exists, I gratefully acknowledge their assistance over the years.

As you already know, I advise a careful review of the foods you have been eating, identifying high calorie sources. The next step is to find lower calorie foods to substitute for those. Pennwalt called this *How to Get Rid of the Calories You'll Never Miss*. To show you how I want your mind to work, here is part of that section of their booklet.

Table 7

How to Get Rid of the Calories You'll Never Miss
BREAKFAST

FROM:		TO:		SAVI
1 scrambled egg	120	1 boiled egg, soft or hard	78	42
2 slices bacon	100	1 slice bacon	50	5C
2 slices white bread	126	2 slices gluten bread	70	56
2 pats butter	200	2 pats light butter	100	100
4 oz orange juice	50	4 oz orange juice	50	0
2 cups coffee w/sugar		2 cups coffee w/0-cal sweetener		
(2 lumps) & cream (2 tblsp)	220	& nondairy cream (11 cal/tsp)	22	198
TOTAL CALORIES	816	TOTAL CALORIES	370	446

[Even better, substitute a 1-inch strip of lean ham for the bacon and omit the butter entirely.—WBP]

MID-MORNING SNACK

FROM:		TO:		SAVI
1 cup coffee w/sugar (2 lumps)		1 cup coffee w/0-cal sweetener		
& cream (2 tblsp)	110	& nondairy cream (11 cal/tblsp)	11	9
1 small Danish pastry	140	2 low-cal cookies (25 cal each)	50	9C
TOTAL CALORIES	250	TOTAL CALORIES	61	189

LUNCH

FROM:		TO:		SAVI
Hamburger	350	Hamburger	350	0
1 slice apple pie	370	Low-fat yogurt	130	240
8 oz whole milk (3.3% fat)	150	Reduced/low fat milk (1% fat)	100	50
TOTAL CALORIES	870	TOTAL CALORIES	580	290

MID-AFTERNOON SNACK

FROM:		TO:		SAVE
12 oz Pepsi regular	150	Low calorie cola	2	148
1 custard (4 oz cup)	140	2 low-cal cookies	50	90
TOTAL CALORIES	290	TOTAL CALORIES	52	238

DINNER

FROM:		TO:		SAVE
6 oz meat loaf w/4 tblsp gravy				
(41 cal per tblsp)	844	6 oz club steak, lean, broiled	120	724
½ cup mashed potatoes	123	1 medium potato, baked	100	23
½ cup green peas	72	12 spears asparagus	40	32
2 slices buttermilk bread	220	1 slice Italian bread, light	45	175
2 pats butter	200	No butter or margarine	0	200
Tossed salad w/1½ tblsp		Hearts of lettuce w/low-cal		
blue cheese dressing	150	salad dressing	35	115
Iced plain layer cake	290	1 cup low-cal whipped dessert	123	167
1 cup coffee w/sugar (2 lumps)		1 cup coffee w/0-cal sweetener		
& cream (2 tblsp)	110	& nondairy cream (11 cal/tblsp)	11	99
TOTAL CALORIES	2009		474	1539
TOTAL CALORIES FOR DAY	4235		1536	2699

TOTAL CALORIES SAVED FOR DAY: 2699 CALORIES!

Now you're saying (or thinking):

- "No one eats that much for dinner." [They don't?]
- "I can see ways to save even more calories." [Good.]
- "I would either skip the morning and afternoon snacks or munch on a fruit or vegetable." [Excellent.]

Of course, some one sat down and made up a hypothetical high calorie day, then showed you how to make it a low calorie day. Here's the important point: *This is how I want your mind to work!* By figuring out and following your own calorie-saving strategies, you will lose weight. *Do this every day!*

Keep this in mind as you reduce calories. As we said before, if you can reduce your intake by 500 calories a day, you will have a net caloric deficit of 3500 calories in 7 days. If you lower your intake by 700 calories a day (which is not hard to do, especially if you have been taking in alcohol calories, non-diet soft drinks, desserts, or other high-calorie items), you will accumulate a 3500 calorie deficit in 5 days. *Each time you accumulate a deficit of 3500 calories, you lose one pound.* This means that you can lose one pound a week (at an average of 500 calories a day) or one pound every 5 days (at 700 calories a day). For most people, that is the expected rate of weight reduction, 4 to 6 pounds a month.

The Pennwalt booklet listed many examples of intelligent substitutions that could lead to saving hundreds of calories. I'll reproduce part of the list, shortened and edited slightly. Again, this is how we want your mind to work:

Table 8

Calorie-Saving Substitutions

FOR THIS		SUBSTITUTE THIS		
BEVERAGES	CAL.		CAL.	SAVED
Milk, whole, 8 oz	150	Skim milk, 8 oz	66	84
Prune juice, 8 oz	170	Tomato juice, 8 oz	50	120
Colas, regular, 12 oz	150	Diet sodas	1	149
Coffee w/cream & 2 tsp sugar	90	Coffee w/0-cal sweetener	0	90
Cocoa, all milk, 8 oz	235	Cocoa, milk & water	140	95
Chocolate shake, 8 oz	350	Lemonade, w/Equal	70	280
Beer, 12 oz	146	Liquor, 1½ oz, w/soda	100	46
BREAKFASTS	CAL.		CAL.	SAVED
Kellogg's Frosted Flakes, 1 cup	160	Puffed wheat, 1 cup	60	100
Eggs, scrambled, 2	220	Eggs, boiled/poached, 2	160	60

BUTTER & CHEESE

Butter on toast	170	Apple butter on toast	90	80
Cheese, Swiss,		Cottage cheese, non-fat,		
1 slice (1 oz)	110	curd, ¼ cup	45	65
American, 1 slice	110	Cottage cheese, same	45	65

DESSERTS

Carrot cake, cream				
cheese iced, 2-inch	390	Cantaloupe, medium, ¼	50	340
Cheesecake, 2-inch	200	Watermelon, ½-inch slice	60	140
Chocolate cake w/icing	340	Sponge cake, 2-inch	120	220
Pound cake, 1/8 cake	250	Plums, 2	70	180
Cookies, assorted,				
3" diam., one	120	Vanilla wafer, dietetic	25	95
Ice cream, strawberry,				
½ cup	130	Strawberries, 8 medium	45	85

PIES

Apple, (1/7 of 9" pie)	345	Apple, fresh, medium	80	265
Blueberry, 1 piece	290	Blueberries, frozen, ½ cup	40	250
Cherry, 1 piece	355	Cherries, whole, ½ cup	45	310
Custard, 1 piece	280	Banana, small, one	85	195
Lemon meringue, 1 pc	305	Lemon gelatin,		
		sugar-free, 1 cup	10	295
Peach, 1 piece	280	Peach, whole, one	35	245

POTATOES

Fried, 1 cup	480	Baked, 2½ inch diam.	100	380
Mashed, 1 cup	245	Boiled, 2½ inch diam.	100	145

SOUPS

Creamed, 1 cup	210	Chicken noodle, 1 cup	110	100
Bean, 1 cup	190	Beef noodle, 1 cup	110	80
Minestrone, 1 cup	105	Beef bouillon, 1 cup	10	95

VEGETABLES

Baked beans, 1 cup	320	Green beans, 1 cup	30	290
Lima beans, baby,				
boiled,1 cup	229	Asparagus, 1 cup	30	199
Corn, creamed,				
canned, 1 cup	200	Cauliflower, 1 cup	30	170

SNACKS

Fudge, 1 oz	115	Vanilla wafers, dietetic (2)	50	65
Potato chips, 10				
medium, 1 oz	150	Pretzels, 10 small sticks	35	115
Corn chips, BBQ, 1 oz	160	Oyster crackers, 45 pc	70	90
Peanuts, salted, 1 oz	170	Apple, fresh, medium	80	90

Gets boring, doesn't it? But there are lessons to be learned from this list. One is to substitute fruit or a vegetable for higher calorie foods, even if not similar (apple for peanuts). Another is to substitute almost anything for fats (apple butter instead of butter on toast, baked potato instead of fried, berries instead of pies with shortening in their crusts). Still another: cutting the size of the portion in half saves 50% of the calories.

This refers, of course, mainly to eating at home. In general, that's the best way to limit calories and lose weight. This worked well in the old days, when one family member was the breadwinner and the other (almost always the mother) stayed home, was there for the children when they came home from school, supervised after-school snacks, prepared the meals and made sure the menus were not designed to foster obesity. One of the major lifestyle changes leading to the Obesity Epidemic has been the dual-income family, with both parents working daily, leaving little time for a spouse to tend the house and children, as well as preparing healthful meals.

Now let's talk about the way Americans really eat and see why the Epidemic flourishes.

Fast Foods

A recent survey said that average Americans eat at restaurants four times a week. It didn't say so, but this survey result must reflect the American public's love affair with fast food franchises. I would separate them from real restaurants, where you sit down and are served (sometimes even with tablecloths), but apparently the survey didn't. Let's talk about fast foods first and real restaurants later.

Allan Borushek's *Calorie Counter* gives figures for the foods of 101 fast food and restaurant chains, using their tricky brand names for products. From these, I will use just McDonald's, Burger King, and Wendy's to show how calorie-rich their most popular offerings are. I will also list a few counts for Arby's, Kentucky Fried Chicken, Subway, and Taco Bell. Lest we neglect pizza, we will look at Pizza Hut and at frozen pizza at home.

Just a reminder: *All caloric values are approximate*, but for our purposes we need to speak of them as though they were exact. In this book, the stated number of calories have been taken from a number of sources, not just the little book I advised you to buy and use. That's why not every figure will be what you see in whatever guide you use. Don't let that bother you.

The burger chains. Table 9 shows the caloric values the burger chains furnished to Borushek for some of their most popular products. Instead of giving values for their sandwiches, Wendy's listed sandwich ingredients separately: bun 160-190 (plain or Kaiser), hamburger patty 100 or 200 (2 oz or 4 oz), American cheese 70, lettuce 15, mayonnaise 30 (1½ tsp).

As you look over this table, what's the first thought that crosses your mind? "If I am restricting my intake to 1200 calories a day, every one of these items has too many calories!" Right? *Right!* Do you see why the answer to "Do you want fries with that?" should *always* be "No, thank you ?" *Yes, you do.*

I looked over the entire food lists for these chains, seeking an item with less than 200 calories. There are none, except in their breakfast menus, and we have already discussed that matter. Two scrambled eggs are listed as 160 calories. But avoid the sausage or bacon items. (Too much fat and too many calories.) A plain English muffin gives Egg McMuffin a total of 290 or sausage McMuffin 360 calories. Hash brown potatoes add 130; hot cakes with margarine and syrup add 600 calories! Even a low-fat apple bran muffin contains 300 calories, plus 100 for each pat of butter if you use a spread.

Table 9

Caloric Contents of Items Commonly Ordered at Burger Places

Food Item	McD's	B K	Wendy's
Big Mac or Whopper	590	680	580*
Big Xtra or Double Whopper	710	920	---
Big X w/cheese, DW w/cheese	810	1020	---
Fries, small	210	230	---
medium	450	400	420
large/Biggie	540	590	470
super/Great Biggie	610	600	570
Hamburger	280	340	270+
Cheeseburger	330	360	310+
Quarter-pounder/Whopper Jr.	430	400	390
McD Fish/BK Big Fish	470	710	470-570
Chicken (nuggets)	430 (9 pc)	340 (8 pc)	230 (5 pc)
Sauces, packet	45-60	35-120	45-250

*Big Bacon Classic   +Junior

Watch the sauces and salad dressings! A single packet of McNugget sauce (all flavors) has 40-60 calories: light mayonnaise (40), barbecue or honey (45), honey mustard or sweet and sour (50), hot mustard (60). Salads vary from garden or grilled chicken

Caesar salad (100) to chef salad (150), but look at the packets of dressing: red French reduced calorie or Thousand Island (130), Caesar or honey mustard (150), or ranch (170). Only vinaigrette (30) is low in calories — as I told you previously.

I suppose you could make a case for stopping in for a garden or grilled chicken salad (100), with one packet of vinaigrette dressing (30), but when was the last time that anyone anywhere did this? And what are you going to drink? If you choose milk, you pay 99 cents for 8 ounces. Milk is much less costly at home, where the salad you make is better also. Of course, a milkshake is out (360 for *small* chocolate, strawberry, or vanilla). Of course, if you order something silly like McFlurry Oreo (570) or Butterfinger (620), you have blown half a day's allowance of calories in one fell swoop!

So your best plan is to *avoid the burger places entirely.* This is important, not only for your own weight reduction and maintenance but also for being a role model and educating children in correct eating habits.

The 2002 lawsuit against fast food chains by a fat opportunist with heart disease was, at first glance, ludicrous. No one forced him to eat fast foods at all, much less to eat them frequently. On the other hand, the chains relentlessly advertise their products, especially the double or triple burger items, as though this is the way people should eat. And, of course, they teach their employees to add that seductive question, "Do you want fries with that?"

You will now very likely shun these fast food giants. But what about fat people who don't read this booklet and who continue to add more blubber by their fast food habits? Try to educate and persuade them. *Buy them a copy of this book.* And if they choose not to learn calories and lose weight, give them each a big forehead sticker that says "STUPID." Not that it's necessary. Their obesity and their failure to correct it says the same thing.

Arby's. Let's move on to Arby's, whose lunches I first enjoyed when I moved to Arizona (1974) and there was an Arby's across from the building in which I worked. What could be wrong with some lean roast beef, thin-sliced, in a bun, with a little sauce to flavor it? The Borushek *Calorie Counter* surprised me. My regular roast beef sandwich (350), Arby Melt or Arby-Q (340, 360), and Beef 'n Cheddar (480) are all higher in calories than I had expected. So are their 6-inch sub sandwiches: French dip (490), hot ham and Swiss (530), Philly beef 'n Swiss (700). Fries, of course, are outlandish, as are Jalapeno Bites (330), mozarella sticks (650), and baked potatoes (500 to 650, depending on toppings). Surprisingly, potato cakes (2 pieces) are lower (250).

Arby's does have a "light menu," from garden salad (70) to roast turkey deluxe (260). Chicken sandwiches go from grilled chicken deluxe (450) to chicken bacon 'n Swiss (610). Chicken Finger Snack (580) and Chicken Finger 4-Pack (880) are even higher if you add even one packet of a sauce or dressing:

Table 10

Caloric Values of Sauces in Fast Food Places

Arby's Sauce	15	Honey mustard	50-130
BBQ dipping sauce	45	Horsey Sauce	60
Bleu cheese dressing	300	Mayonnaise	90
Buttermilk ranch	360	Ranch	250
Honey French	250	Thousand Island	130-260

Caloric contents for sauces and dressings are much the same everywhere, so you can use these numbers wherever you encounter similar items.

So much for Arby's. Their sandwiches still taste good. They may have a place on your weight-*maintaining* program but not on your weight-*losing* program.

Kentucky Fried Chicken. KFC's longstanding entrees have these caloric values for one serving:

Table 11.

Calories in Various KFC Offerings

	Original Recipe	Extra Crispy	Hot & Spicy
Breast	400	470	505
Drumstick	140	195	175
Whole wing	140	220	210
Thigh	250	380	355

Their widely advertised popcorn chicken contains: small (360) or large (620). Hot wings, 6 pieces (470) and honey BBQ, six pieces (610) are both too high. Side orders such as BBQ baked beans (190), biscuit (180), coleslaw (240), potato salad (230) could further add to the total—if you eat them. We still haven't found low-calorie fast food, have we?

Subway. This chain has used a long-running ad campaign featuring a customer's weight reduction by eating only low-calorie subs. Allan Borushek's *Calorie Counter* lists these values for popular subs: ham (260), roast beef (265), roasted chicken (310), Subway Club (295), turkey breast (255), turkey breast and ham (265), and Veggie Delite (200). Subway offers the best selection of fairly low calorie foods among the fast food places, if you simply can't stay away from all of them and eat fewer calories at home. But don't be tempted by their "classic subs, 6 inch." These range from steak and cheese (360) to meatball (500).

From Subway's list of "classic salads, without dressing," a few have 200 calories or less: steak and cheese (180), Subway Seafood & Crab with light mayo (200), or Subway Melt (200). The only salad dressing low in calories (2-ounce packet) is fat-free Italian (20). Others are fat-free ranch (60) or French (70), each in two ounces. Vinegar (1 cal per tsp) remains the best choice.

Taco Bell. Does Taco Bell help us with any low calorie choices? Not really. Unfortunately, the same high caloric values apply to the same Mexican food items at home.

Lowest breakfast items are a country or fiesta burrito (270 or 280). Add hash brown nuggets (280) and you have nearly half of your day's allowance (1200). All other items are 380 to 480 calories per item.

Their burritos range from chili cheese (330) to 7 layer (520), their chalupas from chicken or steak (400) to Santa Fe beef (440). Gorditas contain from 290 to 610 calories, tacos from 190 to 380. There are so many variations that you will have to look them up in your own copy of the Borushek *Calorie Counter*, which I trust you have purchased by now. Taco Bell specialties, as well as nachos and side orders are also too numerous to list here. Suffice it to say that most of them add a lot of calories.

Pizza Hut or Frozen Pizza at Home. What can we say about what has practically become America's national dish? Let's start by remembering this: anything that starts with doughy crust and cheese all over it contains significant calories. You can reduce the content some by ordering thin crust and, of course, avoiding crusts stuffed with cheese. Also resist those "free" breadsticks that some pizza places offer. They aren't free of calories, adding about 140 each if plain, 180 in cheese sticks, and 30 calories or more for dipping sauces.

For toppings, Pizza Hut's thin crust (one medium slice) lists cheese (200), Veggie Lover's (190), pepperoni (190), sausage (290), Meat Lover's (310). Be sure to double or triple these figures if you have two or three slices. If you eat more than that, you are unlikely to reach your weight-losing goal. There's no such thing as a pizza that's low in calories, regardless of where you buy it.

You may also want to look at two pages of caloric values for frozen pizzas that you can bake at home. The list makes your mouth water, but all begin with dough and cheese. It is difficult to justify including pizza in a 1200-calorie program.

If abstaining entirely from fast foods and pizza is more than you can bear and you are thinking of abandoning your weight reduction program entirely, let's at least mention a possible compromise. [You don't have to do it, you know, just because we mention it.] If you do a good job of limiting calories all month and are losing one pound or more every week, allow yourself just once, at the end of the month, to indulge in one fast food "fix." All that can happen if you only stray from your low-calorie course on that infrequent occasion is to delay your eventually reaching your ideal weight. It's your life, your joints, your self-esteem in that improved appearance, so you decide.

However, the psychology is backwards if you seemingly "reward" yourself with a high-calorie meal. In truth, *you reward yourself every day* that you *limit calories* and create a deficit toward losing another pound, toward reaching your slim-trim weight.

If you work and ordinarily grab your lunch at a fast food place, here's another thought. Recently I heard an economist on a TV talk show say, "If you take your lunch to work with you every day instead of buying it, in your working lifetime you will save $150,000." So there's something to be said for brown bagging your lunch, at least part of the time. You can take a giant step toward long-term weight control by planning and carrying low-calorie lunches.

This decision can be a major part of your plan to reduce by 500 to 700 calories a day less than your previous intake and thus lose one pound every five to seven days. It's your choice, and this would be a good one. And who knows? You might set an example for co-workers, even start a movement toward helping them also to limit their calories and save all that money, just as you are doing.

Real Restaurants

I draw the line between fast food places and real restaurants in this way: fast foods can be handed to you through a drive-in window or as you stand up to a counter; real restaurants are those in which you sit down at a table and are served, sometimes even on a tablecloth! Where does this leave cafeterias? They belong in the "real restaurant" category, except that you directly choose your foods, based on the food's appearance and appeal when you are hungry, then carry them to your table.

Restaurants usually give you too much to eat. Only a few gourmet chefs give modest-size portions, basing their appeal on cooking excellence and visual presentation. But how many restaurant meals eaten in the US are this type? Very, very few. Far less than one percent. Characteristically, restaurants have always served their patrons too much, so the word-of-mouth recommendations would be, "You *can't believe* how much they give you to eat!" Some brag about this, or even advertise it. Denny's widely advertised Grand Slam Breakfast (795; 1030 with syrup or margarine) could be breakfast for two. Not only that: Denny's lists seven breakfasts of 1,000 calories or more! My informed readers will avoid such bargains. And they will never patronize any "all you can eat" restaurants, no matter how inviting this may sound.

What can we do to avoid restaurant pitfalls? First, be aware, as you will be for everything you eat, of the caloric content of the foods you order. Of course, you can't really know until you see the *serving size* (the first thing you look at on the label, remember?). But you *are* in control. Always order the *petit* filet instead of the larger steak. Use what you know about potatoes to order the lowest in calories (usually a baked potato, with no sour cream, cheese, butter or margarine). (Salt and pepper work just fine.) Or bargain with the waiter for an extra vegetable instead of potato or rice. Be sure to avoid the exorbitant calories in the tempting desserts, of course.

The other strategy is to *eat only half of the calories* in the dinner the restaurant serves. If two persons share the meal, you accomplish this purpose. The tendency is to give a little more to the member of the duo who can better afford a few more calories, and that's all right. Or, if you order a complete dinner all for yourself, make it a point to *eat only half* of the main calorie sources and take the rest home with you. That's why restaurants have containers for this purpose. That way you get two meals instead of one, which is how to reduce the cost of eating out.

Watch out for uncounted calories. It's OK to nibble on the tray of rolls or freshly baked bread while waiting for your entrée, but be sure to avoid spreading them with some of the butter that came with them. Don't be fooled into dipping your roll into a plateful of olive oil (45 per tsp; 120 per tblsp, ½ ounce). Be sure you know about how many calories are in the bread or rolls, and don't multiply it by eating several servings.

At the Mexican place, don't fill up on the chips placed on the table while you're waiting. Recognize their fat content and how the calories add up. Corn chips average about 150 calories for each serving, but what is the serving size? For most chips, just *one ounce!* Do you realize how few chips that represents? Eleven unbroken chips on my postal scale! Multiply 150 calories by the number of ounces a hungry person consumes before a meal, while commenting on whether the salsa today is hot or medium, oblivious to the fact that even the tangiest salsa doesn't reduce the chips' caloric content.

It boils down to this: Enjoy eating at a restaurant, but don't leave your calorie-consciousness at home. Be aware of caloric values, as you are at home, and use the special strategies listed here. Order wisely. Share the meal or take half of the food home with you. Avoid piling up unnoticed or uncounted calories in bread, rolls, or chips. Avoid fried and french-fried things, as you do everywhere, as well as butter and margarine. And, of course, no rich desserts. These strategies can help you to enjoy a restaurant meal without impairing your weight reduction program.

Bon appetit!

Miscellaneous Stuff You Should Know
Before We Go On

Smoking and weight reduction. If you are a cigarette smoker, you should *quit smoking immediately!* If you don't, please paste that big "STUPID" sign on your forehead and wear it until you do quit. Smoking a pack of cigarettes a day *doubles* your risk of heart attack. If you are also obese, the increased risk is even greater. For many years, smoking has been the biggest cause of preventable deaths. Nowadays obesity is rapidly catching up and may soon become the number one cause of preventable deaths. Obviously a combination of obesity and smoking is deadly. When you quit smoking, the doubled risk of heart attack soon returns to a normal risk. Quitting also stops adding to the risk of emphysema, today's leading cause of disability, and of lung cancer and bladder cancer.

It is important to quit smoking and start your weight reduction program at the same time, rather than fighting first one habit and then the other—and probably failing at both. With your carefully planned dietary program, you will avoid the slight weight gain that otherwise commonly occurs soon after kicking the cigarette habit.

You *can* quit smoking *now*, just by deciding to do so and doing it. Here's how I know that no addiction prevents you from making this most important step toward better health in your future. Suppose you are in the hospital, with oxygen running, the ECG monitor working, and an IV drip in your arm. Your doctor walks into your ICU room with your reports, which show that your chest pain had indeed meant a heart attack. He would say, "Yes, it *is* a heart attack. *You must never smoke another cigarette!*" You would say, "Don't worry. I'll never smoke again." And you would keep that promise to yourself. My question has always been, *why wait for the heart attack?* Stop now and cut your risk in half!

What about vitamins? A daily program of 1000, 1200, or 1500 calories can furnish all the vitamins an adult needs if you base it on protein and include daily citrus fruit or juice, yellow foods, bread, milk, and a good variety of foods in general. However, an inexpensive multiple vitamin supplement will assure an adequate supply of essential vitamins. If you have 30 pounds or more to lose (which means that your weight-losing phase will require at least five or six months), a single multivitamin tablet or capsule each day is probably a good idea. Ask your pharmacist for the least expensive (generic) multivitamin he sells. *Avoid* vitamin preparations that contain *iron.* (The reasons are too detailed to explain here.)

What about salt? For the average person who has no medical condition that makes salt restriction necessary, eating a moderate amount of salt does no harm. Here's a useful rule for most people: Do not use the salt shaker at the table. Salt in cooking is fine if not overdone, but keep your hands off the shaker at the table. It's not a bad idea to add this caution: Avoid things with salt that you can see and taste (salted nuts, salted crackers or pretzels, salted margarita glasses).

If a person has borderline high blood pressure or a family tendency, there are just two things she can do, trying to keep from developing full-blown hypertension, which requires medication: lose weight and avoid salt at the table. Of course, there are medical situations that require salt restriction: congestive heart failure or fluid retention from any other cause. Your doctor will decide whether you need such restriction, possibly with diuretic medication as well. This book makes no attempt to advise you in regard to any medical matters except weight management.

Calcium. Osteoporosis occurs in both sexes, although it has received more attention in women, owing to its exaggerated progression after menopause. Two factors are important in lessening osteoporosis over the years: calcium intake and weight-bearing exercise. These really should begin in adolescence and be a part of the rest of one's life. As time goes by, milk-drinking and exercise have lessened in our population as a whole. However, it is never too late to begin doing the best we can from here on. Along with this, we need to guide children and adolescents into proper habits now, rather than allowing them to substitute carbonated beverages for milk at meals.

A woman needs at least 1000 mg of calcium a day until menopause and 1500 mg a day after that. We have emphasized this over the years but have paid little attention to a man's calcium needs, which we can assume to be about the same. An eight-ounce glass of milk contains 300 mg of calcium. A slice of cheese ("singles") contains 212 mg. Some brands of orange juice are now fortified with calcium; read their labels to learn how much.

If one's intake of calcium in foods falls below the amounts mentioned, a calcium supplement is in order. The labels should clearly spell out the calcium content, sometimes called "elemental calcium." (We aren't interested in how many mg of calcium *citrate*, calcium *carbonate*, or calcium *gluconate* each tablet contains, just its *calcium* content.)

During my years of practice, I sometimes recommended Tums as a source of calcium. Each tablet contains 500 mg, so I suggested thinking of a day's requirement, after menopause, as three Tums. Each time a patient takes 500 mg from milk, cheese, or orange juice, she may omit one tablet. Tums can be dissolved in the mouth or chewed and swallowed. They are easily carried in a purse and, yes, they *are* antacids, capable of relieving heartburn. The company also makes Tums EX (750 mg) and Tums Ultra (1,000 mg), but the 500 mg size is usually more convenient unless you never use any calcium-containing foods.

The body absorbs calcium poorly. Its absorption improves if vitamin D is added; 20,000 units twice a week is enough. Some calcium supplements contain vitamin D.

For a long time the traditional advice was for post-menopausal women to take estrogen (hormone replacement therapy, sometimes abbreviated as HRT), not only to relieve menopausal symptoms but also to stimulate bone formation, as the body's own hormones do during child-bearing years. To produce this effect, a woman had to take more than a small dose of estrogen; a smaller tablet or skin patch does not offer this osteoporosis-lessening effect. For a while it was believed that oral HRT also had a protective effect against coronary heart disease. That's the way it stood when I wrote my 1998 book (*Cholesterol Control Without Diet! The Niacin Solution*).

During 2002, an impressive report changed this situation. Not only did HRT *not* reduce the risk of heart attack; in fact, it *increased* this risk, as well as that of other blood-clotting disorders. In addition, it *increased* the likelihood of several cancers. These included not only uterine cancer (a risk that adding a second hormone, progesterone, had seemed to eliminate) or breast cancer (which had always been a worry for many HRT recipients), but also several other types of cancer!

This caused turmoil in the debate about "HRT or no HRT?" The best option now seems to be to treat any symptoms of menopause with the smallest effective dose of estrogen (the skin patch, maybe) for only as long as the symptoms persist. I never pushed women to take HRT if they were concerned about the increased possibility of breast cancer. If a woman was using enough calcium, with regular weight-bearing exercise, I encouraged her to get along without HRT and avoid that cancer worry.

I have never been a fan of diphosphonates, approved in recent years to lessen bone destruction and perhaps increase bone formation when tests show reduced bone density. Fosamax is the most widely prescribed. Notice carefully the side effects the next time you encounter an ad for this drug. But again, this is a matter for you and your doctor to discuss and decide.

Weight-bearing exercise helps prevent loss of calcium from bones, presumably because the up-and-down jostling of the bones stimulates bone-forming cells. Walking is ideal from all standpoints. Half an hour a day should be plenty. More about exercise later. (Yes, we'll talk about it even though it plays such a small role in weight loss.)

Vegetarian eating. Here we will borrow part of a discussion from *Cholesterol Control Without Diet! The Niacin Solution.* Vegetarians adopt this preference for various reasons. If the reason has anything to do with atherosclerotic disease [narrowing of arteries by cholesterol plaques that can cause heart attacks, strokes, or other circulatory problems], some facts from an expert, Mary Enig, PhD, may lead vegetarians to reconsider.

After acknowledging that vegetarians tend to have significantly lower cholesterol levels than others, Dr. Enig calls attention to several little-known facts. Both male and female vegetarians have *lower HDL (good) cholesterol*, an undesirable situation. Male vegetarians have *lower* mortality from coronary heart disease than male non-vegetarians, but they have *equal* death rates from all causes. Female vegetarians, on the other hand, have *higher* coronary mortality than female non-vegetarians and *much higher* all-cause mortality. Furthermore, autopsy studies have shown that vegetarians have *just as much atherosclerosis* as non-vegetarians, even though vegetarians have lower serum cholesterol levels. Conclusion: if the goal is prevention of heart disease and other atherosclerotic diseases, a vegetarian diet is not the answer.

Dean Ornish, a San Francisco MD-author, has been an advocate of a strict vegetarian diet as part of a complicated program to reduce heart disease. His small "Lifestyle Heart Trial" assigned 28 patients with coronary disease to a treatment group and 20 patients to a usual-care group. The diet provided fruits, vegetables, grains, legumes, and soy bean products without caloric restriction. No animal products were allowed for the treatment group except one egg white and one cup of non-fat milk or yogurt each day.

Stress management techniques included stretching exercises, breathing techniques, meditation, progressive relaxation, and imagery. Patients were asked to practice these techniques for at least one hour a day. Exercise, usually walking, was prescribed according to baseline treadmill performance, advising a minimum of three hours a week in sessions of at least 30 minutes.

Twice-weekly group discussions provided social support to help patients adhere to the lifestyle program. These were led by a clinical psychologist, who "facilitated discussions of strategies for maintaining adherence to the program, communication skills, and expression of feelings about relationships at work and at home."

During the year of the trial, the experimental group had reductions in total cholesterol (24%) and LDL (bad) cholesterol (37%). HDL (good) cholesterol did not change in either group. X-rays of coronary arteries showed a little reduction in cholesterol deposits in the experimental group and a little average progression in the control group. Five men in the control group also showed slight regression of atherosclerosis. They were said to have exercised more often and for longer periods, plus eating fewer calories and less cholesterol than the control patients who showed progression of their arterial narrowing.

Ornish and his colleagues correctly questioned whether such comprehensive lifestyle changes could be sustained in larger populations of persons with coronary disease. They said, "The point of our study was to determine what is true, not what is practicable." My reaction as a practicing physician was that this bizarre program would appeal only to a very few persons. The key word in their title is "lifestyle." Who wants a week full of such time-consuming interventions that it leaves little time for really living? Patients whom I knew would almost unanimously have chosen a program that allows a normal American diet and requires a few pills each day, with knowledgeable medical supervision.

What about soy? This question sometimes comes up when I do radio talk shows or speak to groups about cholesterol control. For a short answer, I again turned to my friend, Mary Enig, PhD, author of *Know Your Fats*, a recent book for scientists, dietitians, and other professionals. She counseled, "I usually try to remind people that soy is filled with phytoestrogens, which act like female hormones. ["Phyto" means *plants*; estrogens are, as you probably know, female hormones.—WBP] In children and in men, soy foods disrupt their hormone production if taken in excess. Soy has unpredictable effects in women. Vegetarian mothers produce male infants with hypospadias at significant rates; this has been traced to soy food intake. [Hypospadias is a developmental anomaly in the male, in which the urethra opens on the underside of the penis or on the perineum.—WBP] Premature breast development in girls has proved to be related to soy infant formula consumption. Research in Japan reports problems with thyroid function." Thank you, Mary.

"Health foods," "natural," or "organic" foods. Don't waste your money. Products sold in "health food" stores *are not approved by the US Food and Drug Administration (FDA)*. Many are rumored to help age-related memory loss, male impotence, postmenopausal problems, etc. The makers of "supplements" are not permitted to tout their products for such benefits in their labeling, so they label them as a "nutritional supplement" and spread rumors that they help this or that. Usually they don't, and they may pose a hazard by interacting with prescription medications if the patient doesn't think to inform the doctor of these "supplements"—that are really medications, untested and unapproved. Doesn't it make sense that if any herbal "supplement" had any of the desirable effects mentioned above, everybody would know about it and everybody with the medical problem would be taking it? And neither of these is true.

The "natural food" label attempts to take advantage of vague consumer concern about "food additives," which have been rumored as possible causes of various health problems, usually not based on good scientific evidence. Remember these reassuring facts:

(1)   Without added preservatives, many of our foods would spoil easily, allowing disease-producing bacteria to multiply at will. That *would* be a serious problem and there would be nothing vague about the cause.

(2)   As one Harvard nutrition expert has pointed out, there is no evidence that even one human has developed cancer or other serious disorder as a result of food additives.

(3)   The FDA is a very effective agency that investigates alleged problems concerning food additives, as well as other ingredients. It bans any food substance that good scientific evidence shows to be hazardous. My four years in the pharmaceutical industry (1974-1978) convinced me that FDA does an excellent job of safeguarding the American public in regard to both foods and drugs.

Formula diets. It has now been forty years or so since the first pre-mixed, canned formula diet appeared. Its name, Metrecal, soon became a household word. For a while it was trendy, as it seemed to offer an easy way to trim weight: drink three cans of Metrecal (several flavors, 300 calories per can) a day—and nothing else! The product seemed to offer an easy way to manage the calorie problem (900 a day), at least part of the time. The drinks had enough protein and carbohydrate to sustain a person seeking to lose weight. Metrecal was quite popular and sold rather well for a few years. At one time the Metrecal manufacturer released a report saying that they had followed a group of subjects who *had no food except Metrecal for two years!*

Of course, competitors brought out similar products. SlimFast was the only name I could think of offhand that is still available, but the Borushek *Calorie Counter* lists 42 different brand names, some with several variations. About a decade ago the Slimfast TV ad campaign included then baseball manager Tommy LaSorda and several rotund football coaches from the NFL. They stood as a group, posing for "before and after" pictures. I would like to line them up now and see whether their canned formula diet programs were *permanently* successful. We both know the answer to that one, don't we?

The obvious problems with this approach are that it really is not a way of life for long-term use and that it doesn't teach anything that will work for you over the long haul. You are better off with my approach, learning the caloric contents of every food you eat and then using this information to advantage as you steer a low-calorie course through life's temptations. *You know that you can do it. Go ahead and show the world*

The Fast Food Lawsuits

At first glance, the first 2002 lawsuit against fast food chains by an opportunistic obese man was ludicrous. No one forced him to eat fast foods at all, much less eat them frequently. However, the chains have always advertised their products, especially the double and triple burger items, as though these were normal parts of a sensible diet. They also lure you with 99-cent prices (or even less) for some of their mainstays and add their oft-repeated question, "Do you want fries with that?

Predictably, other persons contacted the plaintiff's attorney and filed lawsuits of their own against the fast food giants. Class action lawsuits are inevitable and may be in the works by the time you read this. As the attorney pointed out, at one time it seemed silly to sue tobacco companies for health consequences of smoking. However, such lawsuits eventually resulted in numerous rulings against Big Tobacco, with huge dollar settlements. They also led to bans on tobacco ads on TV, to mandatory *anti*-tobacco ads about health hazards, and to laws in many communities (as well as the entire states of California, Delaware, Florida, and New York) against smoking in the workplace and all public places.

It is impossible for a book to be up to date with ongoing news like the fast food lawsuits. The same New York attorney went on to sue McDonald's and two Bronx franchises in behalf of two fat teenagers, on the basis that the chain's billion-dollar ad campaign encourages children to eat their unhealthful foods with-out telling their parents (or anyone) about the health hazards of the excessive weight the foods promote. At this writing a federal judge has thrown out the teenagers' lawsuit, declaring that people are responsible for what they eat and their attorney failed to show that McDonald's engaged in deceptive practices to conceal information about their products. The attorney said he plans to re-file the suit.

McDonald's attorneys wrote, "Every responsible person understands what is in products such as hamburgers and fries, as well as the consequences to one's waistline and potentially to one's health, of excessively eating those foods over a prolonged period of time." In my opinion, this overestimates the intelligence of a large segment of the American people. Did you realize the devastating numbers of calories in fast food items before reading them in this book? And you are a bright person who reads books.

McDonald's cannot deny that they have lured children—and parents with them—into their outlets by adding cheap toys and child-oriented packaging ("Happy Meals"). Other chains have had similar promotions, based on trendy movies and the like.

An earlier *New York Times* story on the teenage lawsuit said that "if their lawyer…makes it to trial with the suit, he hopes to turn it into a class action on behalf all New York children under the age of 18 who claim health problems they say resulted from eating at McDonald's." Our local newspaper editorialized: "Would anyone put McDonald's cuisine in the 'healthy' category. It's doubtful. McDonald's is a place you go when *the kids have pestered you too much* or you *have to grab something on the run.* No one recommends it as a steady diet."

Unfortunately, parents often decide to take this easy way out and grab something on the run, even if the kids aren't actively pestering them. The editorial assumption gives the public more credit than they deserve for having the calorie information and applying it intelligently, day in and day out. That's why this book is necessary, providing information in easily readable style and telling the offenders (and there are many) to *get tough with that excess fat* by consistently using what you have learned about weight control.

Getting Tough With Food Advertising. Here's what needs to be done. *There should be a federal law* requiring fast food places to display, in large numbers, the number of calories in every advertised food product. On TV, the number would have to remain as long as the picture shows or the voice-over talks about the product. An ad for a Big Mac [590] or Burger King Whopper

[660] could be an educational experience. KFC honey BBQ chicken [6 pieces, 607] would be an eye-opener. So would a calorie count for Denny's Grand Slam breakfast (795, 1030 with syrup or margarine) or other "Slams" (710-1250).

The caloric values should also be displayed on large menu signs inside the restaurant and at the drive-in window as well. As the attendant takes the order, whether at the counter or at the window, the caloric value for each item would be displayed to the customer on a computer screen.

An unlikely possibility would be for the employee to state the caloric value of each item when reviewing the order. (Of course, the values would be on the computer right in front of him.) It would go something like this: "Welcome to Jack-in-the-Box. Your order, please." [The customer orders.] "All right, sir. That's a bacon cheeseburger (760) and chocolate shake (630). Do you want fries with that? (350 regular, 430 jumbo)."

But this law must not apply only to fast food places. Calorie information should be required for *all food ads* in TV, radio, or print media, as well as for *cooking shows* and *cooking segments* on TV. All *printed menus* should have to list calories for each item. So should *drink machines* [Pepsi, regular, caffeine-free, 12 ounces, 150; A&W root beer, 12 ounces, 180]. Some people just prefer to remember what the dentists tell us, that a can of regular soda contains the equivalent of 10 to 12 tsp of sugar (15 calories per tsp). That may be easier to remember.

A *beer ad* would have to give the calories per 12 ounces [146 regular, 100 light]. *Bars* would be required to display usual calorie counts for a shot (1½ ounces) of liquor and *measure only that amount* in their drinks. (No overpour, unless they publish an exception to this usual rule as their policy. Then still measure, and report the calories in the measured amount!) They would also display caloric contents for *mixers* [90 in 12 ounces of 7-Up or ginger ale, and even in bitter Canada Dry tonic water], as well as a list of mixers with no calories at all.

Of course, to bring this into proper perspective it would be necessary to teach the public that to lose weight one probably needs to limit to about 1200 calories a day, give or take a little. And tell them to be guided, either by this arbitrary standard or by whatever daily target level the doctor recommends.

All this should become federal law. Impossible? Not at all. Remember that tobacco advertising has been completely removed from TV. Hard liquor ads have been banned from TV for decades, and there has recently been talk of forbidding all alcohol advertising before 10 p.m. *You can help* by organizing a "Contact your Congressmen" movement, urging those who represent you in Washington to sponsor the calorie information bill I advocate. *Copy this chapter and send it to them!* (See page 129 for a sample letter.) If revealing caloric contents were required, food chains and restaurants *would try to outdo each other with low-calorie fare*— which is one of the goals of *The SG Report.* (See next chapter.)

On another matter, restaurants have also been blamed for an observed increase in the portion sizes served and eaten at home, according to a 2003 report from University of North Carolina. They found a trend toward bigger portions in restaurants, packaged foods, and even in recipes. Then they reasoned that this increase in restaurant servings spurred larger helpings at home as well, which plays a significant role in the Obesity Epidemic. People get the idea that the huge portions (super-size offerings at fast food places, as well as "all you can eat" specials are examples) are normal, appropriate amounts. Larry Lindner, executive editor of the Tufts University Health and Nutrition Newsletter, added, "Once a person has become accustomed to eating larger portions, it's difficult to go back to more modest meals."

That's why we have urged you to *take charge of your life*: buy small, use smaller plates, reduce serving sizes to 2/3 of your earlier helpings, and limit the amounts you eat, at home and in real restaurants. (Remember our plan to take about half of restaurant food home?) By limiting serving sizes, you take a significant step toward reducing your daily intake by those 500 to 700 calories that will result in your losing a pound every 5 to 7 days.

While the early lawsuits were pending, McDonald's made two announcements that seemed designed to improve their public image and perhaps distract the public from the legal proceedings. The first news release said that they were reducing the trans-fatty acid and saturated fat content of their US cooking oils. They did not claim that such changes would benefit their patrons, just that "We have learned that topics like food, health, and diet are very important to the public, as well as to health experts, *yet there are conflicting viewpoints.*"

Two issues are involved. The first is the controversy about whether TFA's (trans-fatty acids) present a hazard to health, by producing or worsening atherosclerosis—narrowing of arteries by plaques of cholesterol. TFA's are produced when liquid vegetable oils are solidified to convert them to spreadable margarines. I have always taken a neutral position on this matter but have pointed out that there is really no convincing evidence that TFA's lead to atherosclerosis. There is merely the inference that margarine use in this country, during and since World War II, coincided with the increasing occurrence of coronary disease.

A leading anti-TFA spokesman over the years has been my good friend, George Mann, MD, a retired cholesterol researcher at Vanderbilt. He recently admitted to me that the sinister TFA effects just mentioned have not been substantiated by good studies. There certainly have been no studies comparing the effects of TFA restriction with their unlimited use to see whether there was any difference in coronary events and deaths—nor could such a study ever be conducted. That was good enough for me. Don't clutter your thinking by worrying about TFA content of oils and table spreads. *Cholesterol Control Without Diet!* tells you to go ahead and eat butter, unless you prefer the flavor or cost of margarines. The McDonald announcement about changing oils looks like an image-improving ploy, as the lawsuits were (or are) pending.

What about saturated fats? There *is* some evidence over many years that unsaturated fats (liquid vegetable oils, mainly) slightly reduce blood cholesterol levels. However, a government-sponsored study a few decades ago showed that even highly motivated subjects, with excellent dietary teaching and specially prepared foods, would not follow diets with enough fat restriction to make any difference. Furthermore, it made little or no difference if they did.

Another important study in California (Stanford and UCSF) found that the Step One AHA diet, recommended for everyone, reduced cholesterol by a trivial amount. The AHA Step Two diet (recommended for high-risk persons) lowered total cholesterol by only 5% (still very little). However, it reduced *good* cholesterol as much as *bad* cholesterol—an unfavorable situation. My book, *CCWD!,* points out that diet does so little for cholesterol that we might as well say it does nothing. To control cholesterol properly, one must *change the body's cholesterol factory.* This can be only be accomplished by medications, of which *niacin does everything right* for the cholesterol profile. The widely advertised *statin* drugs do only one thing well (reduce bad cholesterol).

Changing McDonald's cooking oils by reducing TFA's and saturated fats does *not* change their caloric content. We should *avoid all fats used for deep frying—french fries or anything else.* In March 2003 McDonald's announced that they might not make these changes in the fats used for deep frying. Stay tuned.

In January 2003, before the first lawsuits had been thrown out by a federal judge and after their first-ever quarter that showed a financial loss, McDonald's issued a memo telling their managers that they were going to change the flavor of Big Macs. Network news reports said that, when asked for details, the company told the media, "We are playing to win and will take necessary action" but gave no further explanation. A fast food executive speculated that they might tamper with the flavor by adding cayenne pepper or similar ingredient, then test-market the changed product. And by the way: Do you want fries with that?

The Surgeon General's Call to Action

To Prevent and Decrease Overweight

and Obesity, 2001

That's the title of an impressive report issued at the end of 2001, just before David Satcher, MD completed his service as Surgeon General of the United States. This excellent report is a short booklet (60 pages, 5½ x 8½) that is quite readable. It teaches, "Our ultimate goal is to set priorities and establish strategies and actions to reduce overweight and obesity. This process begins with our attitudes about overweight and obesity." It spells out a list of five "overarching principles," to which the report is committed. I like the first two:

- Promote the recognition of overweight and obesity as major public health problems.

- Assist Americans in balancing healthful eating with regular physical activity to achieve and maintain a healthy or healthier body weight.

In a pair of maps of the US, the report compares the prevalence of obesity in 1991 and 2000. Here are the percentages of obesity (defined as 30% overweight or more) in 1991 and 2000:

Table 12

The Surfacing of an Epidemic: Prevalence of Obesity

in American Adults (% of States in Each Category)

Year	No Data	<10%	10-14%	15-19%	20%+
1991	3	8	36	3	0
2000	0	0	1	28	21

In case the numbers are hard to follow, this is what they say: In 1991, 36 states had 10% to 14% of their population falling into the group that was obese (more than 30 pounds overweight). In only 8 states did fewer than 10% of their citizens report their status as more than 30 pounds overweight, and no states had more than 20% of their residents in the obese category.

Look at the same figures for 2000! Only one state (for the curious, it was Colorado) had only 10-14% of its persons in the 30-pound overweight (or more) category. None had fewer than 10% of residents who were obese. In 28% of states (up from 3% nine years earlier) 15-19% of the residents were now more than 30 pounds overweight. By then 21% of states had more than 20% of their population in the obese category. Is it any wonder that those studying the advance of the Epidemic of Obesity are appalled by its rapid progress?

This survey used *self-reported* height and weight to calculate obesity. Self-reported data may (and probably does) *underestimate* the prevalence of obesity, the report warned.

Here's one more table about the Epidemic, and then I won't bore you further with numbers. After all, the number that really matters is *one* (you), or a small number, representing your family members that are too heavy and need the help this book can give.

Table 13
Overweight and Obese Persons in U.S.
at Several Points in Time

Years	Healthy	Overweight	Obese	Total Fat
1976-1980	53%	32%	15%	47%
1988-1994	44%	33%	23%	56%
1999	39%	34%	27%	61%

While the percentages in the overweight category (less than 30% above ideal weight) have remained about the same, look at the increase in obese people (more than 30% over ideal weight)! In the past two decades, this percentage rose from 15% to 27%. At the same time, 14% moved up from *healthy* weights to the *overweight* category, keeping its percentage in the 30's.

The figures vary a bit, depending on the survey that developed them. It now is usual to say that, of the 61% of US population with too much weight, 31% are in the obese category and 30% merely overweight. There's no way to keep up with the exact figures. Just by looking around, you can see obesity taking over our society. It is tragic to realize how these fat people are impairing their health, shortening their lives, and destroying their quality of life. And they are doing nothing about it.

Those were the last figures available when the SG report was compiled in 2001. Surveys this large take two years or more to complete, which is the reason that available figures lag two years behind the current year, sometimes more. There is not the slightest doubt that the obesity epidemic has continued to increase since then.

Quite properly, the report (which, for purposes of our discussion, I shall shorten to "*The SG Report*"), points out that the Epidemic of Obesity is relatively recent. Government, as well as any right-thinking person, is distressed by the epidemic's rapid increase and the health threat it poses to an ever-increasing part of our citizenry.

The report says, "This approach should focus on health rather than appearance." It recommends not stigmatizing fat people but "addressing overweight and obesity in a positive and proactive fashion."

Health Risks for Fat People. All right—let's focus on health. So far I have mentioned only heart disease and degenerative joint disease as major adverse effects of excessive weight. But look at **Table 14**, borrowed from the *Call to Action*, titled *Health Risks Associated with Obesity.*

Table 14

Obesity Is Associated with an Increased Risk of:

Premature death

Type 2 diabetes

Heart disease

Stroke

High blood pressure

Gall bladder disease

Osteoarthritis (degeneration of cartilage and bone in joints)

Sleep apnea

Asthma

Breathing problems

Cancer (uterus, colon, kidney, gallbladder, postmenopausal breast cancer)

High blood cholesterol

Complications of pregnancy

Menstrual irregularities

Hirsutism (excess body and facial hair)

Stress incontinence (urine leakage caused by weak pelvic floor muscles)

Increased surgical risk

Psychological disorders such as depression

Psychological difficulties from social stigmatization

Do you see anything on the list that you would like to avoid? All of them? No one can argue with that. I still want to emphasize the major health reasons to get rid of excess fat: reducing your risk of heart disease and stroke, of diabetes, and of wearing out your weight-bearing joints. I especially want you to avoid these major intrusions into your life as a healthy adult. You *can* do it! Will you?

Ethnic Groups and Fat. There are disparities in the prevalence of overweight in various segments of the population, based on race and ethnicity. Excess weight is more common in minority groups and those with a lower family income. Rather than burden you with still another table, I suggest that you look back at figures from the American Heart Association (Table 1, page 4). The *SG Report* analyzes the figures further, but it doesn't matter.

$$$ Consequences of Fat. The *SG Report* points out the overall economic consequences of overweight and obesity that you and I seldom think of. The increasing prevalence of excessive weight increases direct costs of medical care: physician visits, hospital and nursing home care. There are also indirect costs, the value of wages lost by people unable to work because of illness or disability, as well as future earnings lost by premature death. According to the SG report, the total (direct and indirect) costs related to obesity increased from an estimated $99 billion in 1995 to $117 billion in 2000. Most of these costs were due to type 2 diabetes, coronary heart disease, and high blood pressure.

Here's a statistic we think of even less. Obese persons earn, on average, about 5% less than those who are not obese. I am not sure who developed this figure, but it was featured on national newscasts in the fall of 2002. They reported that over a 40-year career this amounts to $100,000 less than the average of non-obese workers. This is not a health issue and probably has something to do with social stigmatization, although there may be an element of an obese person's inability to perform some jobs. It's just another reason to get rid of the excess weight. I haven't yet seen any reason to gain or keep the extra pounds, unless you are a Sumo wrestler.

The Solution for All Fat People. The solution to the problem is the same for all groups: *Learn the information in this book and use it!* That is why we have kept the book's cost as low as we can, hoping to encourage everyone to urge their friends to buy and use the book. We hope that employers will buy it in quantity for their employees and that service organizations will decide, as one of their projects, to spread this life-saving information. Anyone can contact Lilac Press regarding quantity discounts.

We hope that many readers will take advantage of our bargain value (fifth book free when you buy four) and share the information with friends and relatives, with the request that these persons in turn pass along books to five more people.

What has government done so far? Government tends to take a long time to analyze a situation, writes a report that defines its next goals, recommends further research, and perhaps, sooner or later, gets around to things people or communities should do. That's the story of the 2001 *Call to Action.* According to its introduction, the report resulted from a series of activities: a December 2000 "Public Listening Session on Overweight and Obesity," a public comment period, and the National Nutrition Summit. Did you ever hear or read of any of these? Neither did I.

The SG report assembled "useful starting points" for individuals and groups, who were invited to use their skills, creativity, and inspiration on the Epidemic. They developed a menu consisting of Communications, Actions, Research and Education shortened to the acronym "CARE." Then they applied these to each of five key settings:
  (1) families and communities,
  (2) schools,
  (3) health care
  (4) media and communications
  (5) worksites.

Some of these overlap. As I review the list and write (early in 2003), I wonder whether anything has yet been accomplished because of the 2001 *Call to Action.* It will be interesting to see whether government will get tough, as it could do, to eliminate some of the abuses that have combined to favor the Epidemic.

For *Families and Communities*, the section titled *Communication* begins with "Raise consumer awareness about the effect of being overweight on overall health." That's what this book aims to do. What has government done so far? Have you noticed anything in your area?

"Inform community leaders about the importance of developing healthy communities." Also "Highlight programs that support healthful food and physical activity choices to community decision makers." What has anyone done so far?

"Raise policy makers' awareness of the need to develop social and environmental policy that would help communities and families to be more physically active and consume a healthier diet." Sounds good, but how would you do that? And yes, exercise is important for other reasons, but let's not fool people into thinking that it plays a major role in weight reduction.

People would differ in their views on what constitutes a *"healthy* diet."* I would say simply *low enough in calories to lose excess weight.* Others would insist that a diet must be low in saturated fat, low in cholesterol, possibly with added polyunsaturated fat, and maybe lots of fiber. Still others might even suggest various other maneuvers thought by some to affect cholesterol or aging. But I have already explained to you that diet has little or nothing to do with your blood cholesterol, that diet only lowers cholesterol during periods of weight reduction, and that diet reduces good cholesterol as well as bad cholesterol, an unfavorable situation. (*Cholesterol Control Without Diet! The Niacin Solution* goes into more detail about how to readjust your body's cholesterol factory if your blood cholesterol pattern is unsuitable.)

Here are some of the reasons I *do not* recommend a government publication titled *Dietary Guidelines for Americans*: It is too complicated and is based, in part, on mistaken beliefs of some of NIH's favorite consultants. Some of these consultants drew up the 2001 Cholesterol Guidelines, which are badly flawed.

---

*The proper word would be *"healthful"* habits or diet. Only a living thing can be *healthy*—except, of course a "healthy" sense of humor.

One chapter in the 2003 edition of *CCWD!*, titled *What's Wrong with the 2001 Cholesterol Guidelines?*, spells out more details.

The Epidemic in Children and Adolescents. Besides teaching persons who are already overweight or obese a new set of habits that will lead to weight control, it is important to prevent extension of the Epidemic into the next generation of children and adolescents. It can be done and should be a major goal. This is a challenge for adults, their children and teenagers, and for health leaders: seeking ways to keep young people from falling victim to the Epidemic and its future consequences.

I especially like parts of *The SG Report's* section on *Communication (Families and Communities)*. Here's one: "Educate parents about the need to serve as good role models by practicing healthy eating habits and engaging in regular physical activity in order to instill lifelong healthy habits in their children." It also advises: "Raise consumer awareness about reasonable food and beverage portion sizes." (My thoughts exactly, as you know.)

Under *Action*, the report encourages community efforts to provide increased opportunities for leisure time physical activity and "to encourage food outlets to increase availability of low-calorie, nutritious food items." To help to combat the extension of the epidemic to children and adolescents, the report advocates that parents "decrease time spent watching television and in similar sedentary behavior by children and their families." This is a worthy goal. How to attain it is not clear, but it obviously will have to be the subject of a huge publicity campaign with widespread support if it is to succeed. It will take time. We need to start now.

Under *Schools*, the report contains some good ideas, like spreading the messages of healthful eating and increased physical activity. Schools definitely should require physical education (We used to call it "gym.") for all students throughout their school years. *It is a disgrace that less than ten percent of high schools require PE in the senior year.* Many require little or no PE throughout adolescent years and may just go through the motions in grade schools. Every school child should be required to have gym periods at least twice a week from first grade through high school! The time should be specified, from 45 minutes to an hour of actual exercise. And intramural sports should be emphasized for the vast majority of students who are not in varsity sports.

I am getting as bored as you are by this review of parts of *The SG Report.* Let's step back and consider measures that could be taken by government, some at the national level, others at the local level—school boards or health departments. Remember that some of the measures that have been legislated against tobacco would, at one time, have been considered out of the question.

Getting Tough About Calories. As already discussed, *there should be a federal law* requiring fast food places to *display, in large print, the number of calories in every advertised food product.* Caloric values should also be shown *on all menus*, including those outside and inside fast food places and real restaurants.

We have noted how such a law would also apply to drink machines, ads for alcoholic beverages, and bars. TV ads for foods, as well as cooking shows and cooking segments on general talk shows would also be compelled to list calories in the same unmistakeable, easy-to-read manner. Foods in cafeterias, *especially those in schools*, should be labeled in the same way.

None of this will happen without heavy and continuous pressure on Congress, and *that will not happen without your efforts.* To make this easier for you, we are including a sample letter to your Senators and Representatives in Washington (Appendix A) that you can use or modify it to your needs. Send a copy of this book with it if you choose to do so. This could have the additional benefit of reducing those expanding Congressional waistlines that are leading to heart attacks, diabetes, and worn-out weight-bearing joints, as in the rest of our population.

The SG Report expresses the hope that restaurants and fast food places will try to out-do their competition by developing and publicizing low-calorie fare. The "Truth in Calories" law would be an important stimulus leading toward this goal. *It will happen if you make it happen!* Be a leader, organizing groups (PTA's, service clubs, whatever group you belong to or can contact) to join you in lobbying for this all-important health reform. The day is here (and overdue) for us, as a nation, to take charge of our lives and provide this help for others to do so as well.

Reducing Calories in Schools. At the local level, let's get the soft drink machines out of the schools. Find out whether your schools have contracted with fast food chains to serve their students. This is a hot issue across the country since the soft drink giants and fast food chains pay schools to help them hook students on their foods. They do this by giving money for band uniforms, sports equipment, digital cameras for photography classes, etc.— luxuries the schools will be reluctant to give up. It's up to parents and others interested in students' health to bring these practices to light, then try to eradicate them. Challenge school boards to join you in fighting to eliminate the sodas and fast foods, replacing them with health*ful* foods *The SG Report* encourages. Good luck!

Of course, for school-based education in healthful eating habits to succeed, students must be kept on campus during the noon hour. In our area, and perhaps yours as well, it is common for high school students to pile into a car and speed off to nearby fast food places for lunch. Too often this practice has resulted in auto accidents, sometimes with loss of life. Besides getting rid of soda machines and fast foods in the schools, closing the campuses during the noon hour should be another goal for caring parents.

While campaigning with your school board, why not prod them to institute gym classes (physical education, if you will) from the grades through high school, thus showing their dedication to a complete program of weight control? We have already discussed this and cannot emphasize it enough. It's your job.

Obese Adults Raise Obese Children. Come to think of it, while writing this book I *have* come across more newspaper columns and magazine stories about the increase in childhood and teenage obesity. Maybe this is merely my increased interest and awareness. I doubt that these writers have written their articles because of *The SG Report.* More likely, they have just looked around them, been impressed by the Epidemic, and seized on the subject for an article. Statistics are easy to come by, and it only takes a few to spice up an account.

The major network news programs have covered the issue with information-laden stories. They have pointed out that each year about 300,000 Americans die from illnesses caused or made worse by obesity. As we have noted, more than 60% of adults in US are overweight (30%) or obese (31%). The networks have noted (as we did, page 7) that black and Hispanic men are only slightly more obese than white men (21.3% and 24.8% vs. 20.8%), but black and Hispanic women have much more obesity than their white counterparts (38.2% and 36.1% vs. 23.2%).

That fat adults are passing their poor eating habits down to their children is a major concern. Children growing up today learn poor eating habits from parents who find it easier to buy fast food or order a pizza than to prepare a healthful, low-calorie supper. The schools teach children to operate a computer at an early age, setting them up for sedentary computer games after school rather than basketball, volleyball, soccer, tennis, and other physical exercise. Children often accompany their sedentary activities with high-calorie snack foods and soft drinks, as do fat adults. Some parents even allow soft drinks instead of milk at meals. Parents *can* control the type of snacks (how about fruit?) in the house and exclude those with more calories. They should do so.

Studies have shown that the amount of TV that children watch is linked to the Epidemic of Childhood Obesity. With unrestricted access to TV, they watch more and do less. The American Academy of Pediatrics (AAP) advises a maximum of two hours of *quality* TV programming a day, but studies show that the average child watches at least three hours a day, not necessarily of high quality.

The AAP's advice to parents: Take the TV out of the child's bedroom, and take the computer out of the bedroom as well. A Harvard study found that 54% of children had a TV set in their bedrooms, and 42% said that their parents set no restrictions on how much they could watch. Those with bedroom TV's viewed for about 3.8 hours a day, compared to 40 minutes less for those who had to watch elsewhere. Children who had no TV in the bedroom and whose parents limited their TV watching spent more time doing homework and reading.

Children who ate dinner with their parents watched about 30 minutes less TV than those who did not. For many reasons, *parents and children should eat dinner together.* This puts the parents in charge of their children's foods and eating habits. Not only can they put into practice the knowledge they have gained about calories; they can also use the strategies I outlined (page 27), the smaller plates, smaller servings, putting silverware down between bites—you remember. Most important of all, it serves as a time for families to talk to each other on a regular basis.

The Harvard study showed that reducing TV viewing by about one-half hour a day led to a reduction in obesity. So did parents' taking an active role in regulating their children's media habits, not only the amount of viewing but also its content.

Dr. Miriam Bar-on, speaking for the AAP, said, "There are plenty of studies that have linked television and video games to violence and violent behavior, substance abuse, [and] altered body image." So *parents, take charge!* Your children's health and psychological adjustment is in your hands!

Social Stigmatization of Fat People. Yes, we will always emphasize health, but it is impossible not to characterize the fat people who comprise the Epidemic in terms some would consider stigmatization. We should not be so sensitive about our terminology that we refer to fat people as *plump, heavy, chunky, chubby, big-boned,* or similar euphemisms. The word is *fat*—as in "I am too fat and I'm going to do something about it." That's what you should be saying to yourself many times a day to bolster your resolution to do the right thing *every time* you make a choice about calories.

Look around you. Isn't the size of many people appalling? Looking at fat people is like watching smokers destroy their health. Do you remember that both groups qualified for the "STUPID" sign, unless they are doing something about it *right now*? If fat people take the view (similar to the stance smokers often take about smoking) that "I'll stay fat, ruining my heart and weight-bearing joints if I want to," they should at least understand that their ignoring such an obvious health hazard sets a bad example for their children or others for whom they serve as role models.

Think of the last time you saw a fat family, perhaps entering a restaurant, or guzzling hot dogs, sodas and/or beer at a ball game. Both parents are fat and getting around slowly, with effort. Could they run if they had to? Probably not, and if they tried, it would better be described as *lumbering.* Some are even entering the group we call *massive* or *morbid obesity*, in which case they waddle. Notice that the older children are the fattest, and the amount of fat declines to the youngest, who may not yet be fat—but you can bet will get there, given more time. The children are oblivious to what is happening to them. After all, aren't Mom and Dad huge? I eat what they put in front of me, in about the same amounts they eat. I guess being fat just runs in our family.

What kind of a friend are you if you let the fat people you know stay that way, instead of giving them the benefit of this book's message? We need to get away from timidity by saying to those fat people we know. "Here's a book that will help your whole family (or Jim, or whoever). It tells the truth about weight control. It is readable and easy to use. I hope it helps you [maybe, *as it has helped us*, if that is so]." For ordering information, see page 136 or look at the web site, www.cholesterolnodiet.com.

Neither we nor you want you to seem to be saying, "You are fat. Here's a book." That's why we include, with each copy, a bookmark that says "Presented with loving concern, knowing that weight control can prevent heart attack and diabetes, while sparing weight-bearing joints." The bookmark says other things and bears an important message to accompany your gift.

Effects of the Epidemic in Our Society. At one time there were a few specialty stores (Lane Bryant comes to mind) that featured clothes for oversize women. Now they still exist, but every clothing store shows, on its racks, the effects of the Epidemic of Obesity. My wife tells me that the women's racks have very few "small" or even "medium" items. But starting with "large" and going on through XL, XXL, "3X," and larger, there are plenty of clothes. Look at the shoppers and you'll see why. Doesn't it look as though more than 31% are obese and more than 30% merely overweight? It does to me.

Some clothing ads are beginning to show models who are overweight, a contrast to their usual bone-thin or normal-size models. Recently I saw a clothing ad, showing that a company was charging more for oversized garments than for those of reasonable sizes. This may not be new. It should have been a policy all along.

Southwest Airlines caught flak when it instituted higher fares for persons beyond a certain girth. Southwest was right to institute this increase in fares. All airlines should follow suit. Airlines will soon begin to charge *by weight* for checked luggage and carry-ons. This policy may be in place by the time you read this. Such charges should be based on the total of body weight and luggage weight, not to punish fat people but merely to be fair to everyone. Fat people *can* take control and achieve healthy weights. This would be another incentive—as if heart disease, diabetes, worn-out joints, and premature death were not enough.

The Surgeon General's Report was a good first step. Now the government must show its willingness to act quickly and decisively. Let's let our voices be heard.

A Review: How Are You Doing So Far?

You haven't read to this point in just one day, have you? That means you have had time to begin to implement parts of the program you will need to reach your ideal weight. Let's review and see whether you are getting into this program. If not, be sure to do whatever it takes to follow the guidelines and start making progress.

Have you started a weight loss diary? It just takes a notebook, your scales, and an official day each week to weigh for the record. Have you taken your photos? That's an important part of getting started. So is measuring your height and weight, finding your BMI, writing it down, and identifying your next goal—the weight that will take you from *obese* to just *overweight*, or from just overweight to *healthy* weight.

If you are in the *morbid obesity* category (more than 100 pounds overweight; BMI of 40 or more), your first goal will be to bring your weight below the BMI 40 level, then aim to escape from the *obese* category into *overweight* and beyond. Yes, there's surgery, which has been high-profiled on TV and in other media, but that is a last-ditch measure, comparable to coronary artery surgery or angioplasty and stent in those with heart disease. We'll have more to say about surgery a couple of chapters ahead, but let's make it clear right now that even morbid obesity *can and will* respond to the calorie control that this book advocates.

Do you have your own copy of Allan Borushek's *The Doctor's Pocket Calorie Fat & Carbohydrate Counter*? It is an indispensable tool, the best I have found. Here's a little bonus that goes with it. You may wish to visit Allan Borushek's website, which is <u>www.calorieking.com</u>. It complements the book with food product updates, as well as extra educational writings. At this writing, they are establishing a newsletter, which should be up and running by the time you read this.

Are you using the strategies that allow you to reduce calories even before you start to count them: smaller plates, 2/3 size helpings, serving at the stove, no nibbling while cooking or clearing dishes, putting silverware down between bites. (I know it may be hard at first, but once you learn this technique it will serve you well.) Do you stop eating when you are *satisfied, not stuffed,* and leave some food on the plate? Do you know the caloric values, at least approximate, of everything you eat or drink? You should, and once you learn these values for the common foods, you will always benefit by applying this knowledge. And *buy small!*

Turn back to the tables that show caloric values for many fruits and vegetables (pages 37-39). It's easy to run through them too quickly and not use them wisely. *Review them carefully.* Think how you can eat twice as many helpings of vegetables each day, to compensate for reduced portions of foods that contain more calories. Also think how good the fruits are and that you can use them as desserts and snacks, replacing high-calorie things you formerly ate.

Are you omitting butter, margarine, and other common items high in calories, including mayonnaise and other salad dressings? Are you thinking in the same terms as *How to Get Rid of the Calories You'll Never Miss*, substituting low-calorie choices for things that formerly ran up the daily totals? Are you remembering that all you must do to lose one pound every five to seven days is reduce previous calories by 500 to 700 each day?

Have you gotten rid of those alcohol calories? Snacks? Candy? Soft drinks? Are you saying to yourself, as many times a day as necessary, "I am too fat and I *am* doing something about it?" Think this way to bolster your willpower each time.

Have you learned that so far there is no such thing as low-calorie fast food and vowed to stay away from places that sell such calorie-rich items? Are you avoiding pizza also? Have you posted a reminder on the kitchen bulletin board or refrigerator, showing calorie counts for fast foods and pizza you once ate?

If you have children, is the family eating together, so you can supervise their menu as well as yours? Are you enjoying that quality time together instead of going off in several directions, which promotes poor food choices by some, especially the younger family members? Do you share your knowledge about calorie control with them? *Do you talk about calories?* Are you about to remove TV and computers from the rooms of children and adolescents, who will then spend more time studying and reading? Have the children who are old enough to understand this book read it yet? They should.

Nothing says that teenagers can't take the lead in reorganizing the family's eating habits. In many instances, children and teenagers learned in school about the devastating effects of smoking and persuaded their parents to give up that deadly habit. Why not do the same with foods and obesity? It works better if a whole family resolves to revise their eating habits by starting to observe low-calorie rules that will lead to normal weights for all. Each can reinforce the others in resisting temptations and following their resolutions to lose weight steadily. They can compare weight-loss diaries, not competitively but in a cooperative effort to reach their common goals. Is your family doing this?

I have great confidence in the intelligence and energy of many teenagers who become activists in some worthy cause and organize to work toward achieving wide-reaching success. To my knowledge, the influence of students on parents in the smoking issue was an individual effort, but mobilizing to combat the Epidemic of Obesity can well be a group effort. I visualize high school "Healthy Weight" clubs, whose members will read this book, hold meetings to share strategies and their own weight control results as well as those of their families if applicable. They could be instrumental in exerting pressure to change school menus (especially if the fast food chains have gotten their products into cafeterias), get rid of soft drink machines, and increase opportunities for exercise.

A faculty advisor might be necessary, but maybe more would get done if the advisor were absent from many meetings, leaving things to the youthful energy and ingenuity of the students. Speaking of that, how about getting rid of obese coaches (usually football). They are not good role models and should be given a deadline to bring weight to a healthy BMI or go back to teaching history or math.

If the answer is "yes" to all of the questions in this chapter, you are learning your lessons well and applying them. If not, now is the time to start doing everything right. *Take charge of your life!* You *will* succeed.

More Miscellaneous Information: Answering Your Questions Before You Ask

Can I "spot reduce" one area? How many times has some one said to herself, "If I could just take off a few inches around the hips?"—or thighs, or tummy. "The rest of me is all right." Is it possible to spot reduce, to lose weight in one area and not others? The answer is *no*. The calorie deficit it takes to lose fat works on all parts of the body where fat is stored. It is not possible to reduce your hips or tummy without your face becoming somewhat thinner and some fat disappearing from other parts of your body.

A machine with a vibrating belt that you put around your hips or abdomen will not remove weight from the area it shakes. A spa employee (usually not a qualified trainer) may tell you that "You don't need to lose weight from your arms; you just need to firm up what you have there." This is one of my pet peeves, as you will see in the exercise section. You can lose fat, and you can build muscle, but merely exercising muscles will not get rid of fatty deposits in any part of the body. Reducing calories will.

Regarding the upper arms, as you get older, you will either have fat flabby arms or thin flabby arms. Thin is better and can be achieved by calorie control.

We inherit the pattern of fat distribution in the body and have no control over it. If you were born with a tendency to heavy calves and thighs (which some unkind persons call "piano legs"), you cannot selectively reduce those parts or change their contours. By calorie control you can lose fat; by exercise, you can build muscle. But the tendency to have a preponderance of weight in the legs cannot be changed. Do your best with calories, then learn to love it. If you are slim and trim otherwise and so fit from exercise that you move around like a much younger person, you will have achieved the possible goals. You will look good and feel good, which your family and friends will appreciate—and so will you.

Waistlines: Where did they go? You remember the waistline. It's that part of the body between the rib cage and pelvis. It is supposed to be smaller than they are, but it's also a place in which both men and women tend to accumulate excess weight, so in many cases it disappears. In the old days, when the Miss America pageant still admitted that it was a beauty contest, they gave the numbers that characterized the bathing beauties' figures: bust, waist, and hips. A 35-24-36 shape was nice. Hips sometimes were no larger than the bust, but a little increase was quite all right. Nowadays, with breast implants, some of the hip measurements must be a bit smaller—but that's another story.

When men put on excessive weight, it tends to accumulate around the waist, variously called a "pot belly" or "beer belly." Of course, this is only a part of the total, all-over fat layer, but it is the most prominent. Where I live, cowboy types often wear their belts below the fat belly, but that doesn't make it any more becoming. The waistline accumulation in women, especially the "apple" shape (as opposed to the "pear") starts by making the former waistline into a straight-line block joining the ribs and pelvis, then on to a rounded protuberance, even larger than hips or ribs.

All this results first in not tucking in the shirt or blouse, in an attempt to mask the fact that a real waistline no longer exists. Next, in women, is the smock or overblouse to hide the overstuffed midriff even more. Finally, giving up entirely, we reach the mumu, caftan, or sack dress stage, a completely shapeless tent, trying to ignore what's underneath.

For many years my office was next to a leading *bariatrician* (specialist in weight reduction) in Scottsdale. Besides his own expertise, he offered to his patients the services of a dietitian, an exercise physiologist, and a behavioral psychologist. One day I asked him why I saw women trooping into his reception room at five in the afternoon on some days. He replied that he had a fashion consultant from a leading department store come in to talk to the women about their clothing choices as they lost weight. When I asked him what she advised as they lost from size to size, he said, "She tells them to wear a sack dress with a sash that they can tighten as their waistlines become smaller." For some reason I thought I could have told patients the same thing without bringing in the department store representative.

Remember that we included *waist measurement* in your diet diary list, along with a weekly weight record. We have already noted that waist measurement is related to the risk of heart attack. (By the way, I think we can ignore such unlikely reports as the claim that "apple shape" is associated with an increase in breast cancer and that a 30 minute walk each day decreases breast cancer by 40 per cent.) As the scales show that you are losing weight, your tape will also show a smaller waist measurement. Both will reinforce your determination to continue to do well. Of course, as your over-size waist subsides, you are losing fat from the layer under the skin that encases most of the body.

How much weight should I lose? Ultimately you are the one who decides how much weight you want to lose. You probably won't know exactly how much before you start, unless you have been at a trim weight recently enough to know what level is right for you. Remember that your youthful weight, if you were not heavy at that time, is not bad as your ideal weight for life.

From the medical standpoint, I recommend that you *trim all excessive fat.* Don't compromise with extra fat; get rid of it! You will look and feel better. You will have reduced the work load of your heart, blood vessels, and weight-bearing joints, all of which suffer if you stay fat. Be tough enough to go all the way! The last five pounds will be even easier to lose than the first five, because by now you have replaced your old, unsuitable eating habits with better ones.

Is it possible to lose too much? Usually not, in well adjusted adults with no eating disorder. Sometimes an adolescent or young adult, usually female, becomes bone-thin from anorexia (medically, originally called *anorexia nervosa*) or bulimia. These are *eating disorders* that require the services of a specialist because they can result in serious physical impairment or death. They are associated with distorted body image in these low self-esteem girls, who think they are fat, even though they have almost no fat on the entire body.

You will not lose too much if you use the BMI table to find the weight that gets you out of the *overweight* category, into the *healthy weight* group, then proceed to whatever weight lets you look and feel as you want to.

Here's why I say to go beyond the borderline between "overweight" and "healthy" weights to reach *your* ideal weight. Look at these figures:

Table 15

Height	"Healthy"	Overweight	Obese
5' 0"	97-128	128-153	>153
5' 3"	107-141	141-169	>169
5' 6"	118-155	155-186	>186
5' 9"	128-169	169-203	>203
6' 0"	140-184	184-221	>221
6' 3"	152-200	200-240	>240

Source: National Institute of Diabetes, Digestive, Kidney Diseases

I submit that a person five feet tall who weighs 125 pounds is overweight. So are persons at the upper limit of each "healthy" weight range, unless they are well-muscled athletes. So you and your mirror decide on *a new slim-trim goal* after you reach the "healthy" range in the tables.

How shall I handle special occasions? If you are doing a good job of trimming calories day in and day out, you may forego your usual program on a few special occasions: Thanksgiving, Christmas, your birthday, your wedding anniversary, or another special family event. However, special days should be kept to a minimum, not more than five or six days a year. My office booklet always pointed out that anyone who insists on overeating on Groundhog Day, Benjamin Franklin's birthday, and Bastille Day may not be serious about losing weight, as their results will show.

Remember the "special occasion" rule: It's not what you do on those few special days but what you do *day in and day out* that determines your success or failure at weight reduction. You may even surprise yourself, as many of my patients did, by discovering that even though you set aside the usual rules for that special Thanksgiving dinner, you end up having small portions of everything you want and just a taste of that wonderful dessert. Many people have come in to say, "You would have been proud of me," for not heaping a plate full, probably two or three times, as in previous years. When this happened, we both knew that new, better eating habits had replaced the old, unsuitable habits. This performance virtually assured that achieving a trim weight was bound to follow.

Can drugs help? This is a matter for you and your doctor to decide, but my answer would be *no*. Nearly everyone has heard of the harm caused by drugs commonly called "Fen-Phen" a few years ago, leading to their withdrawal from the market. These two appetite suppressants resulted in damage to heart valves in a small percentage of patients who used them, but even a small chance is enough to have FDA order a withdrawal, or for a company to withdraw a drug voluntarily to avoid such an order. Advertising lawyers are still looking for persons who used the Fen-Phen combination, hoping to uncover candidates for lawsuits.

Years ago appetite-reducing amphetamines were marketed freely, most of them by one leading pharmaceutical company that manufactured several preparations in plain tablets and time-release

"Spansules." Eventually, the strong potential for abuse of amphetamines led to regulations controlling the prescribing of these drugs. There are still some similar drugs on the market that suppress appetite and have less stimulating effect than amphetamines, although they have some such effect.

The last clinical trial I conducted in Madison, Wisconsin before moving to Arizona in 1974 involved a comparison of an appetite suppressant with a blank tablet (placebo) in patients who received the same diet instruction and were handled exactly the same way except for the medication. The group taking the "diet pills" lost weight more effectively throughout the study, which continued for 12 weeks.

Because I soon left the clinic at which I had coordinated research studies for 18 years, I had no long-term follow-up on this weight reduction study. There was no doubt that the drug gave its recipients a short-term advantage. However, detailed education, like that in this book, was lacking. This is an important ingredient in long-term success: learning where calories are and using lower calorie foods while avoiding high calorie sources that produced the excess weight in the first place.

Instead of considering any appetite-reducing drug—use of which would necessarily be limited to a fairly short term—I would advise you to learn your lessons well from this book and to apply them for the rest of your life. Your doctor will probably agree.

Do I need medical supervision for my program? Ordinarily your doctor prescribes a diet for you. He may send you to a dietitian for instruction, hand you a printed diet that you probably won't follow, or send you to an organized program. (In my experience Weight Watchers has probably done more good than other plans for obese persons, but their long-term success rate is probably about as poor as all the others because of the same human frailty that allowed all that extra weight to accumulate.) Or you may, on your own, decide to try one of the costly approaches to losing weight—probably to become part of that 98% failure rate.

This book is your dietary prescription. It gives you all the diet instruction you need. It tells you to *get tough* and to plan your own program that *will* succeed. When you do see your medical advisor, be sure to tell him that you have embarked on a weight-losing program. Share your weekly weight diary with him. If things aren't going as well as they should, you may know the reasons. If not, your doctor may be able to help you recognize the flaws and get you back on track. One or two simple adjustments can make a big difference.

Show him this book. If he feels it would be helpful to give (or sell) it to his overweight and obese patients, he can contact Lilac Press regarding discounts on quantity orders.

After I started patients on dietary programs for weight reduction, some of them, feeling guilty about not losing weight, failed to return at scheduled intervals to check on their progress. Some even dreamed up, as an excuse for missing or canceling an appointment (as they told me later): "I knew you would scold me." On the contrary, I have never scolded a patient. Even if your effort was not up to par, I would commend your willingness to try harder in the future—and eventually to succeed.

Surgery for Weight Reduction

Plastic surgery following successful weight reduction.
After a person succeeds in losing a substantial amount of weight (to the ideal weight, we would hope), most people are satisfied with the new slim-trim body that resulted from the calorie-controlling methods this book gave them. For some, desiring further improvement in body shape, there are plastic surgery procedures that can help to achieve the desired appearance. One is a "tummy tuck," removing an apron of excess skin from the abdomen that was once filled with fat. I heartily approve this type of surgery, which should be performed *after* the weight goal has been reached. There's no reason to take off a fatty apron while leaving excess fat elsewhere on the body, including the part of the abdominal wall that is not included in the tummy-tuck procedure.

Another method that has received too much publicity and has been overused is *liposuction,* for which some plastic surgeons have coined the term "body sculpting." The important fact for people to learn and remember is that liposuction is for *thin persons* who have an area that remains too bulgy, even after they have lost weight effectively on other parts of the body. A good example is a woman who still has "saddle-bags" after becoming trim elsewhere. Liposuction helps her appearance, if she cares. Possibly "love handles" that persist after successful weight reduction could qualify as well, but they are so common in persons at trim, healthy weights that a person should be happy to ignore them. Unlike the tummy-tuck candidates, these areas are optional, and many successful weight loss patients elect not to have cosmetic surgery, being satisfied with the improved silhouette they have achieved by a sound, calorie-control program.

Liposuction is painful and is associated with extensive bruising, the appearance of which startled even me, a doctor with decades of experience, the first time a patient showed it to me. Think twice before requesting liposuction.

Gastric surgery for massive (morbid) obesity. There are a number of surgical techniques that involve making the stomach smaller and sometimes connecting it to a part of the small intestine, so as to by-pass part of the intestine's absorbing surfaces. Surgery should only be considered in persons with *morbid obesity.* (Morbidity, as a medical term, refers to disease or impairment, as opposed to death, or mortality.

Morbid obesity can be defined in two ways. Some say it means more than 100 pounds over the ideal weight. The other definition is a *BMI more than 40.* The latter is the easier definition. Usually you can spot a morbidly obese person at a distance, laboring to get around.

Morbid obesity is a tragic extreme that not only has the cardiac and joint complications caused by lesser degrees of obesity; it actually poses an imminent threat to life. Such a person *could* actually take charge of things, follow the principles in this book, and lose all of the excessive weight. However, the striking results shown on TV in high profile persons who have had stomach surgery, together with the known threat to life, make gastric (stomach) surgery an important possibility. More and more doctors now refer their patients with morbid obesity to surgeons trained in operations to reduce stomach size and perhaps to bypass part of the intestine as well.

Three leaders in this field, from Louisiana*, warn that "Obesity is a complex disorder with multiple causes that include genetic, environmental, psychologic, and metabolic factors. The obese state is not solely the result of gluttony and sloth. Ultimately, morbid obesity is a complex disease process that requires the collaboration of a wide range of health professionals, including nutritionists, mental health workers, internists, and bariatric surgeons, for optimal management."

*M. Whitten Wise, Louis F. Martin, and J. Patrick O'Leary, in *Current Surgical Therapy, 7th edition,* edited by John L. Cameron, MD.

Detailed pre-operative evaluation is necessary to decide whether a patient is suitable for gastric surgery. Most programs require patients to fill out dietary assessments and psychosocial questionnaires. They meet with nutritionists, psychologists, and exercise physiologists. Usually the exercise expert supervises a limited treadmill evaluation. The Louisiana surgeons say that patients who can complete one mile on the treadmill are less likely to develop complications after operation than those that are not as well conditioned.

Psychologic evaluation identifies significant depression in more than 40% of persons with morbid obesity. Many of them are given antidepressant medication. In addition to laboratory studies as part of complete medical evaluation, prospective surgical patients have studies to rule out gallstones or liver abnormalities. If the history suggests sleep apnea, a disorder most likely to occur in obese persons, sleep studies are also included.

The Louisiana surgeons consider patients for surgical evaluation if they are ages 18 to 60 with a BMI over 40, or with a BMI over 35 and "an appropriate co-morbid condition." This would include problems such as heart disease, high blood pressure, diabetes, significant cholesterol problems, or painful degenerative joint disease in weight-bearing joints. There are few persons with morbid obesity who do not have one of these conditions. If they are young enough not to have them yet, they are surely on their way. In deciding on the operation, the surgeons take into consideration the patients' dietary patterns, preoperative weight, and "most important, their desires."

Hospitals need special facilities if their surgeons are to operate on morbidly obese patients: larger beds, wheelchairs, and toilets.

There are two basic types of stomach operations. The older is *vertical banded gastroplasty (VBG)*. It is the outgrowth of many

partitioning procedures done in the 1970's and is one of two operations endorsed by a panel at NIH (National Institutes of Health) in
1991. By placing a row of vertical staples in the stomach,
reinforced by sutures and plastic (Marlex) mesh, the surgeons
reduce its size to a 20 ml or smaller pouch. Unbelievably, this is
only half of a shot glass!

Weight loss has not been as great as with bypass
operations, described below. Possible complications include ero-
sion of the mesh into the stomach, worsening of acid reflux into
the esophagus (heartburn), persistent vomiting if the stomach's
outlet narrows, and possible leaks. Current teaching says that one
patient in 200 dies during or soon after surgery. This figure may
improve with more widespread use of laparoscopic procedures.

The other type of stomach surgery, which seems to be more
popular nowadays, is *gastric bypass*, combined with a procedure to
reduce stomach size. The technique cuts off the upper part of the
stomach, leaving a much smaller sac, sometimes described as "the
size of an egg." (This is about the same as the 20 ml stomach in
VBG.) This pouch is then connected with the middle part of the
small intestine, thus bypassing much of the intestine's absorbing
surface.

Like other operative procedures such as gall bladder
removal, these gastric operations can be performed laparo-
scopically, using multiple small incisions and equipment that
allows the surgeon to operate on the abdominal organs through a
scope that projects their images on a TV screen. Most gall bladder
operations and some other procedures are now done by this type of
technique, which shortens the time of recovery and of hospital-
ization. For surgery on the stomach in morbidly obese persons,
this surgery requires five to seven small incisions.

Laparoscopic surgery is well suited to gastric surgery for
obesity. Open operation in morbidly obese patients requires large
incisions, and even with forceful retraction it can be difficult or im-

possible to obtain adequate exposure. Also a large incision leads to complications from restriction of lung expansion, plus more wound complications.

An operation called *adjustable gastric banding (AGB)* is especially well suited to laparoscopic techniques and has become popular worldwide. The surgeon places a band around the upper part of the stomach and brings a tube to the outside, through the abdominal wall. The patient follows a liquid diet for four weeks. After two months, small amounts of liquid (as little as ¼ to ½ of a teaspoonful!) are added at a time, adjusting pressure on the stomach according to weight loss, x-ray studies, and the patient's tolerance.

Results of ABG appear to be comparable to those of VBG, plus offering progressive weight reduction after two years. Surgeons are still learning better ways to perform laparoscopic procedures, so results will undoubtedly improve further.

Postoperative care is complex, including breathing into a machine for better lung expansion, using an injected anticoagulant, daily physical therapy, chewable vitamins, medication to lessen development of gallstones, and vitamin B_{12} injections. Patients must be seen frequently and encouraged to continue in weekly support groups, which they started in the preoperative period.

I have not included diagrams of the various operations. It is up to the surgeons and their teams to teach their candidates before these procedures. In my judgment, surgery should be undertaken only as a life-saving procedure in an older morbidly obese person. Recent news stories have touted stomach operations for younger patients, including teens and even younger ages. If still in practice, I would use great caution in young persons. Long-term results of these stomach procedures are not known. Young persons are better candidates for proper calorie control and exercise.

Surgeons caution that their surgical colleagues, internists, *and patients* should be realistic about expected goals. The goal of bariatric surgery is to induce and maintain permanent loss of *at least half* of the preoperative excess body weight. The widely publicized examples of weight loss to nearly normal levels in high-profile persons in TV or other entertainment may not be what the average patient will achieve. In all aspects of medicine, it is foolish to be impressed by percentage results: per cent of cholesterol reduction or of body weight. What really matters is *whether the goals of treatment are achieved.*

The goal is not only to lose a certain amount of weight but also to reverse or markedly improve the various problems caused or worsened by the massive weight. Realistically, about *70% of patients reach a loss of 50% of their excess weight.* They may still be overweight, but their diabetes, high blood pressure, or abnormal cholesterol profiles may return to levels that do not require treatment. (Fortunately, there are good medications to treat these conditions.) Even though destruction of joint cartilage by excessive weight will not be reversed, marked weight loss should lead to improvement in symptoms, especially in hips .and knees. (Back pains don't respond as well.) Surgical replacement of weight-bearing joints should not be considered in morbidly obese patients but can be safer and more effective after significant weight loss.

The down side of gastric surgery, besides one surgical death in each 200 patients, includes post-operative complications, the very uncomfortable "dumping syndrome" (known for decades, following partial removal of the stomach), and possible late complications as well. *Not all patients lose weight after gastric surgery, and some of those who do lose will gain it back!* All in all, the morbidly obese patient should think long and hard about using the lessons this book teaches instead of deciding on surgery. Better yet, just as we can prevent many heart attacks and strokes by treating abnormal risk factors, let's *prevent* morbid obesity in the first place, using these methods of calorie control.

Oh, All Right---
Let's Talk About Exercise

A Fitness Maneuver. Remember my telling you that exercise burns relatively few calories? If I walk on the treadmill for 30 minutes at 3.5 miles per hour and a 2% grade, the digital readout tells me that I have burned *just over 100 calories*. If I ride 5 miles on the LifeCycle, which takes about 14 minutes, the readout shows *only 77 calories*.

In fairness, here's a bit of good news for heavier persons. I weigh about 155 pounds, and the treadmill's computer calculates my caloric expenditure based on this weight. A heavier person burns more calories from the same amount of exercise, so one weighing 200 pounds would use *223 calories* from the same half-hour walk. Do not avoid exercise just because it uses relatively few calories, compared with what you can easily save by knowing food values and being tough.

Regarding exercise, the important thing is not to say to yourself, "I have been *so good* with exercise that it doesn't matter if I have that piece of cheesecake." It *does* matter. A piece of Sara Lee French cheesecake (1/6 of a cake) contains 350 calories, and others are comparable. If I add one slice of bread, at 100 calories, I add about what I burned in five miles on the bike.

Although exercise is not a weight-losing maneuver; it *is* a *fitness* maneuver. As such, it is an important part of a program to reduce weight. A person who is fit is a better walker, and that's the way we get around in this world. As we age, those who walk regularly with vigor do not become weak and lose their ability to walk well. They retain strength in their legs, which makes them look and feel younger than they are.

What is fitness? Fitness is not just the absence of disease. That's *wellness*, a term that makes me shudder because it's a sales tool that is overused in our society today. Fitness is a *positive* quality attained by regular exercise of the *aerobic* type. That is the kind of exercise that makes the heart and lungs work harder for a sustained period of time. The term *aerobics* was originally coined by longstanding exercise advocate Kenneth Cooper, I believe. Unfortunately, it has been corrupted to mean jumping around in time to music, one of many instances in which we have lost a perfectly good word to popular usage. Isn't that what you think of when a person says, "I am going to my aerobics class?"

What exercise do you need for fitness? And how much? Do you remember the best-selling book that proclaimed *All I Ever Needed to Know I Learned in Kindergarten*? There is a parallel here. We could say, "All you ever need to do for fitness you learned at about age one." To be fit, all you need to do is *walk*. You must walk long enough, briskly enough, and regularly enough to meet your own fitness goal. Each of these ingredients deserves brief explanation.

The **duration** of each session should be about 30 minutes. Measure your sessions by the clock, not by the mile. As time goes on, you become a better walker and cover more ground in your half hour. The goal is to exercise your legs, heart, and lungs at whatever pace you can maintain comfortably for that length of time. Longer sessions are fine, but avoid other variations if you can. Splitting the session into two periods decreases its value somewhat but is still better than nothing. However, you can easily understand that six five-minute periods (or, to carry the example to the extreme, 30 one-minute periods) would not be as beneficial.

Avoid the temptation to give yourself credit for exercise on the job, in housework, in the swimming pool, or on the golf course. At best, these add a "plus" to your program but are usually not sufficiently intense and sustained to replace part of your walking program. Later we will mention a few activities that do qualify.

The **intensity** of the exercise should be whatever brisk pace you can continue comfortably for 30 minutes. Don't wear yourself out in the first five or ten minutes and be unable to finish a session at a decent pace. Your legs, heart, and lungs benefit most from endurance exercise, not quick sprints.

Find a pace that is brisk, yet comfortable. An exercise walker should look as though he is in a hurry, not dawdling along and certainly not stopping to chat with friends or to window-shop, if walking in a mall. Walking, because it is *weight-bearing*, is the type of exercise we all need to reduce osteoporosis. Also, to the extent that exercise may help to reduce stress, walking is the only type you really need.

Before going further, let's dispel the myth that we need to drive the heart rate up to a certain level to make cardiovascular exercise worthwhile. This is simply not true. If it were, everyone taking a beta-blocker for blood pressure or heart trouble would be getting no value from just about any exercise, because the drug blunts the usual increase in heart rate. Pay no attention to the pulse-counting myth as you proceed with your walking program.

Regularity of exercise sessions is important. The best program is to walk every day. Build the exercise session into your scheduling, giving it top priority. If seven days a week is a problem, plan to walk six days a week. That's one day off each week for good behavior. Five days a week isn't as good as six or seven but is better than nothing. Less than five days a week is not a regular exercise program.

If you feel too tired to walk after a hard day of work, *walk anyway*! You will feel better, sleep better, and perhaps walk off some of those tensions that made you feel tired in the first place.

Why not run? *Running or jogging is harmful.* Don't forget that. Tell your friends: **running is harmful!** It damages weight-bearing joints (ankles, knees, hips, even low back) by speeding the degenerative process that thins the cartilage lining these joints. This is especially true in the knees, because of the forceful impact of each running step.

A person who weighs 150 pounds jars about three square inches of knee cartilage with most of his body weight with every running step. That's about 50 pounds per square inch. Think of putting your thumb nail (about one-half square inch) on a solid surface and dropping 25 pounds on it—repeatedly, as in running.

Repeating thousands of running steps regularly is a sure way to abuse the knee cartilage and cause premature aging of the joints, with eventual stiffness, pain, and swelling of various degrees. This injury to joint cartilage does not occur with brisk walking, since both feet do not leave the ground at the same time.

Walking exercises more muscles than jogging. The number of calories burned and the value to the heart and blood vessels is about the same for walking as for jogging or running—especially when you consider that the runner may miss weeks of exercise each year due to exercise-related injuries: shin splints, painful heels, sore and swollen joints, aggravated low back problems, and other joggers' ailments.

There was a time when national panels of exercise experts recommended running or jogging. However, in 1993 the Center for Disease Control and Prevention, along with the President's Council on Physical Fitness and Sports, announced a new set of guidelines. Since then they have advised 30 minutes of *moderate* physical activity just about every day, instead of 20 minutes of *strenuous* activity three to five times a week. In other words, they now advised *walking* instead of running. Why? Probably because most Americans were not following the old recommendations.

In 2003, a group assembled to develop *dietary* guidelines decided to expand their responsibility by issuing a statement that the previously recommended 30 minutes of exercise was inadequate and that *everyone should exercise 60 minutes every day*! Give me a break! Most people aren't heeding the old idea of 30 minutes of daily exercise. Don't pay attention to this recommendation if you should see it. No one else will.

On the other hand, a person who is walking at least 30 minutes each day is certainly allowed to add more exercise in this or another form. You may decide to step up the pace at the end of your session, maybe just for the last minute at first but more as time goes by. Using stairs instead of the elevator at work may help if you do this frequently. It's good exercise for the large muscle in the front of the thigh, the *quadriceps*, an extremely important muscle as we age. You decide whether it is worthwhile it to park a distance from the entrance at work or from the store to which you are going, walking briskly as you enter and exit. You may also think of other measures that work for you.

What about other forms of exercise? First, let's make sure there is no misunderstanding about what I mean when I say, "For fitness, all most people need to do is walk." This does not mean that choosing to *add* another type of exercise is wrong.

Sometimes a doctor will prescribe another type of exercise to treat a specific condition. Needless to say, this lies outside the scope of my policy statement about not needing any exercise except walking. Of course you should follow the doctor's advice!

Some people may not be able to walk well enough to gain benefit from it. They may decide, possibly with the doctor's help, to select another form of exercise that they can do. But beyond that, if a person decides on another form of exercise that is really not necessary, let's at least acknowledge that they are doing this for another reason (often *vanity*), not for fitness, as previously defined. For competitive sports, the reason may be enjoyment.

What types of exercise do you *not* need for fitness? Well, first of all, you do not need to pull on your designer leotards and go to the corner "fitness center" to jump around in time to music, probably also going up and down on that little step. (We have already noted that many call this "aerobics," ignoring the fact that walking is the perfect aerobic exercise.) I prefer to call aerobic exercise *endurance* exercise or *cardiovascular* exercise.

Ads for "fitness centers" seem to imply that exercise programs and weight loss are synonymous. By now you know that they are not. Remember, and share with your friends: Those who think exercise will, by itself, lead to weight loss will be disappointed. _Calorie control is the_ only _weight reduction maneuver_. It can be enhanced, but not replaced, by exercise. Walking is as good as (and probably better than) bouncy aerobics, which have the same potential harmful effect on your joints as running or jogging.

This brings us to another kind of exercise no one needs for fitness: weight lifting or other "upper body" exercise. These "grunt and groan" exercises include weight lifting, push-ups, sit-ups, shoveling snow, or pushing a stalled car. [You must understand that parts of my office booklet were written during the years that I lived in Wisconsin.] Except for sit-ups ("crunches), exercises of this type should be avoided by persons with known heart problems or bad backs, including disc problems or osteoporosis. More about sit-ups soon.

Most ordinary persons who enroll in "fitness" programs do not need "upper body" exercises. There's nothing wrong with doing them, but let's realize that one is performing such activities for vanity or for the good feeling that comes with having stronger muscles, not for general or cardiovascular fitness. If a person just wants to build up arm muscles, this can be done at home with one or two inexpensive arm weights.

Certain occupational groups _do_ need upper body strength, including some weight lifting. An overpaid professional athlete will, of course, do whatever work in the weight room that the trainer ("strength coach") advises. Similarly, except that they are underpaid, firefighters and police need the upper body strength to lug their heavy equipment or combat those who resist arrest.

Besides "grunt and groan" exercise, there is another type that may have some value. "stretch and bend." Bending over and touching one's toes (or the floor, if you want to show off) repeatedly is a classic. So is the "jumping jack." One can do these at home, starting with as many as are comfortable and increasing as you can. Like all exercises, it's not how many you do at a time, but rather the fact that you do them daily, that makes any efforts valuable.

Another exercise easily combined with those is the one that helps you to stand and walk with your shoulders back, rather than rounded. This takes me back to Navy days. With elbows bent to a right angle and fists clenched, pull your shoulders back as though trying to touch your elbows together in back. Repeating this daily, as many efforts as you choose, helps the upper back muscles that keep your shoulders erect. One caution, however: a person who is already round-shouldered (like a woman with osteoporosis and a "dowager hump" in the upper back) *cannot* achieve an upright posture to get rid of the hump. It is caused by loss of bone that turns the bodies of the vertebrae into wedges with their narrower side forward, forming an arch instead of a straight spine. Husbands should not urge these ladies to "sit up straight," because they can't.

One attraction of the corner "fitness club" or "spa" (another corruption of a perfectly good word) for some patrons is access to equipment they do not have at home. None of these mechanical gimmicks is really necessary for fitness. The yuppie mentality has led some to buy expensive exercise machinery, in the belief that they will use it regularly. This isn't exactly a racket, but since they charge for something that only a few people continue to use regularly for long periods, it is usually an unjustified expense.

I have read that three out of four persons who join "fitness centers" drop out after three weeks. And only one person in 20 goes regularly to work out. The owners of such establishments must count on this, or they would need places 20 times as large.

Exercises with specific purposes as we age. As we said before, walking is essential to maintain any level of fitness at all.

We can also use some simple at-home exercises for two sets of muscles: abdominal muscles and quadriceps ("quads"), the large muscles on the front of the thighs.

The only way to get rid of a pot belly is to lose the fat by calorie control. However, if you don't have too much fat, you can "pull it in" by tightening your abdominal muscles, can't you? It's a good idea to strengthen those muscles so it will be easier (and can become habit) to tighten them and give yourself a firmer, smaller waistline most of the time. (I recall McLean Stevenson saying to Johnny Carson, years ago, "I took a walk on the beach with Harvey Korman yesterday. Do you have any idea what it takes to hold your stomach in for an hour and a half?")

Sit-ups ("crunches") are worthwhile. We used to call them *sit-ups*, and they are still about the same, even though the trendy term now is "*crunches*." They help most people by strengthening abdominal muscles that we seldom use in daily activities. You don't have to hook your feet under something or have some one hold them down. In fact, to spare your lower back, you should do sit-ups with your knees bent and your feet flat on the floor. A better idea: with knees still up, do this exercise in bed. Do a set before you get up in the morning and another when you get into bed at night. As in all exercise, *regularity* is all-important. This in-bed plan gives you an easy way to remember to do this simple exercise regularly, twice a day.

Some people recommend clasping your hands behind your head. That looks athletic, and you may decide to do it, but it really doesn't matter. Then, using those abdominal muscles, bring your body to an upright or nearly upright position. (I guess the latter makes it a crunch, since you don't really sit *up*.) You can just come up straight, or you can vary the routine by reaching for your left knee with your right elbow and vice versa. It really doesn't matter. What does matter is that you do the exercises regularly.

How many? If you have no trouble doing these exercises, do 30 at a time. You will do more if you want to, but 30 is a good target, done regularly. If you can't do 30 at first, do as many as you can, twice a day. After a week or so, you'll find that you can do more. Increase the number, maybe by 4 or 5 efforts once a week, until you can do 30 at a time. Then do them twice a day.

To strengthen the all-important thigh muscles (quads), I have always advised "*stand-ups.*" As we get older, the thigh muscles become weaker from not being used very much. Older people have increasing difficulty in getting up from a soft sofa or a chair that lets them sink in, bending the knees too far. Some reach the point that even rising from a straight chair is a challenge. A person with forced inactivity from illness or surgery rapidly loses quadriceps strength and needs rehabilitation.

Stand-ups start with sitting in a kitchen or dining room chair, then standing up without using the hands and arms. Repeat these efforts until the front thigh muscles feel tired. Again, there's no point in pushing the number of efforts each time; doing this twice a day, every day, will build strength. You don't have to be old or weak to benefit from this type of exercise. Persons who are more fit can keep the quads working well by regular walking and climbing stairs.

If a person isn't able to stand up from a straight chair, as above, they need help to get started. One is to put a thick phone directory on the chair to raise the starting point. I usually advised the Phoenix phone directory, adding the Yellow Pages if more starting height was needed. You decide what works for you.

Strengthening the quads is so important to keep an older person from becoming feeble that it is worth the effort. Older, weaker persons may need another person to stand by and encourage, or even help if necessary. The payoff is increased strength, better walking, and fending off the disability that can result from quadriceps weakness. Many elderly persons become depressed from their inability to walk well or do other things that they can resume after improving their leg strength.

There's another way to exercise the quads that many may prefer. It can be combined with stand-ups but at different times since each will tire the muscles. There's a machine at the exercise place that does this with weights, but I recall seeing the Physical Therapy Section at the Mayo Clinic (during my training years there) showing patients how to perform this exercise at home without any special equipment.

With the patient seated on an examining table [A high chair or stool works.] so the feet did not touch the floor, they taught the helper to hang the handle of a purse or canvas bag over one foot. With weights in the purse (at home, rocks or other suitable objects) to provide the right amount of resistance, the patient repeatedly and slowly extends the leg straight out and slowly returns it to the down position. The amount of weight should allow the patient to repeat the leg raises 10 to 20 times before the muscles tire. Then repeat the process with the other leg. If possible, try two series with each leg during each workout. If used regularly, this will strengthen muscles so one can do more efforts (repetitions, or *reps*) at each session before tiring. Doing these simple exercises daily can promote greater leg strength and better walking. This, in turn, prevents a worsening situation, with feebleness and disability.

What about outdoor exercise that I enjoy? The way to decide whether an activity measures up as your daily aerobic exercise is to compare it to 30 minutes of steady, brisk walking. Let's consider a few examples.

Bicycle riding for at least 30 minutes a day can fulfill a day's requirement for exercise if you are sure it provides as much exercise to legs, heart, and lungs as a brisk walk. However, here are some warnings. Over the years I had at least three patients who, in falls from bicycles, broke a major bone, either the humerus (upper arm bone) or femur (thigh bone). Another was struck by a car while riding to work.

Always wear a helmet! And be sure your helmet is a good one. As the sign in the bike shop says, "If you have a ten-dollar brain, buy a ten-dollar helmet." Safety-approved helmets are not very expensive. The latest ratings by *Consumer Reports* (summer 2002) showed two "Best Buys" at $35 and $40.

It makes no sense to ride a bike where there are cars. Find safer areas. The SG Report urges communities to provide safe areas for walking; this applies also to bike paths or "multi-use paths." We would hope that communities will respond, but this will take time, even after they get this message, if they ever do.

I don't want to seem entirely negative about bike riding. Done properly, it is good cardiovascular exercise. Since the spine is jostled around somewhat, as in walking, it might be considered weight-bearing exercise to reduce of osteoporosis. A good rider has less risk of injury than a novice or one who hasn't ridden since childhood and isn't very good at it. Brisk walking is better.

My final word on bike riding is this: It is absurd for parents to ride their bikes with small children in child seats, even with helmets on the little ones. This is another example of yuppie mentality! The parents should be walking, with the child in a stroller or other wheeled device—or left at home.

Roller blades (more properly "in-line skates," I suppose) have been a fad among teenagers and adults who aspire to be teenagers again. Like skateboards, an earlier fad still seen occasionally, they have been responsible for breaking many adult bones and for an occasional death in skaters without helmets.

Why any adult would want to skate on roller blades is beyond me. In addition to a helmet, one needs protective equipment for wrists (where the most fractures occur), knees, elbows, and hands. Beginners are always in danger of falls, so fractures are common. When it comes to fitness, the exercise is not as good as walking. There is also a hip motion peculiar to roller-blading that must be wearing out those joints.

Tennis can substitute for walking on a given day if you play an hour of fast doubles or reasonably competent singles. It can give a certain amount of exercise to veterans like me and my tennis buddies, even if we have to say, "Nice shot!" more often instead of running for the hard-to-reach wide shots.

Swimming as exercise is difficult to evaluate unless you swim laps continuously for 20 to 30 minutes. Probably anything short of this can be considered an exercise *plus* but should not replace a daily walk. Persons who are very obese or have painful weight-bearing joints can benefit from exercising in the shallow end of the pool. Just walking from side to side as briskly as you can in waist-deep water is good leg exercise. The water provides buoyancy, lessening the effect of excessive pounds on weight-bearing joints. Any of the funny business termed "water aerobics" (that word again) is likely to be nonproductive, except as a form of walking. Anything involving the upper body is pointless as regards fitness, as previously discussed.

Golf doesn't qualify as endurance exercise because it is not continuous. In the old days, when a golfer would walk the course, carrying or wheeling his own clubs, at least he did some walking, as the pros still do. However, because it was not sustained, it had little or no cardiovascular value. True, the golfer walked some after driving the ball off the tee, but then there was some standing around, waiting his turn for the next shot. As golfers approach the green, walking becomes less and the time standing around becomes longer. During each of these pauses, the heart and lungs return to their normal, non-exercise rates. So much for any valuable exer-cise. And now, golf carts have eliminated walking altogether. I rest my case: golf is not exercise.

Gardening, unless you are walking briskly and con-tinuously with your mower (that day's exercise session if it is long enough), is a mixture of stretch-and-bend and grunt-and-groan exercise that does not provide endurance exercise. At best, garden-ing may be a *plus* but not your full exercise for that day.

At-work walking, unless brisk and continuous for 30 minutes, is just another *plus*. People tend to say, "I'm on my feet most of the time," or "I'm never still," or "I get plenty of exercise doing my housework." They talk like this *before* we teach patients how to evaluate exercise. Walking up and down stairs (especially up) is a *plus*, but only that.

Running sports. It goes without saying that if a person is young enough and in good enough condition to participate in running sports, these can substitute for walking on some days. Soccer, played actively, is ideal for children because it can involve fairly continuous running. Basketball depends on whether you run very much or stand around a lot. You must decide whether the session exceeds a half-hour brisk walk. Speaking of standing around, diamond sports (softball, baseball) involve much standing, with an occasional spurt of energy, but almost no endurance (cardiovascular) exercise. Football is another sport characterized by short spurts of energy, rather than sustained cardiovascular effort. The Kennedys played touch football because they were already in good shape, not the other way around. All in all, soccer for children and basketball, if you do more running than standing, are the most valuable. If you are an adult, walking briskly for 30 minutes a day is the sure way to fulfill your exercise requirement.

What about physical problems during exercise? If anything hurts during exercise, stop. Chest pain, squeezing, or tightness may indicate inadequate blood flow to heart muscle from narrowing of the coronary arteries. Usually it forces one to stop but goes away with rest. *Be sure you* promptly *tell your doctor about this.* You may need an exercise electrocardiogram with an echocardiogram ("stress echo"), or a modified test in persons too obese to walk successfully on the treadmill. Chest pain might be a warning of coronary disease that could lead to a heart attack. Call the doctor *immediately* if the distress lasts longer than 30 minutes, as a heart attack is likely. It will not be helped by denial and delay.

Impaired circulation to leg muscles can cause pain in the calf, thigh, or buttock. Typically a person, after a brief rest, can walk the same distance again. Walking to the point of pain in the legs does not cause harm. In fact, doctors recommend a regular walking program for patients with this type of leg pain.

In a person with narrowed arteries, regular walking, over time, tends to enlarge the detour channels that need to carry more blood if the main channel to a part becomes blocked entirely. This probably explains why heart attacks are less frequent in persons who exercise regularly, compared with those who do not.

One who develops symptoms with exercise is thus alerted to this reduced circulation. He can report the symptoms to the doctor, who will study the situation and advise any necessary treatment. His non-exercising neighbor may have as much narrowing of blood vessels but not know it until his heart attack.

One-third of heart attack victims die of the first attack. In many, *the first symptom of coronary disease is sudden death!* This is why we must discover and, if abnormal, correct the major risk factors for heart attack, stroke, and other artery-narrowing disorders. These major risk factors are *cigarette smoking, high blood pressure, abnormal cholesterol fractions, diabetes, and obesity.* For detailed information about treating these risk factors, read *Cholesterol Control Without Diet! The Niacin Solution*, in its updated, enlarged second edition. (See page 136.) *CCWD!* teaches that *heart attacks are preventable!*

What to do when the weather doesn't cooperate? In many parts of the country it becomes too cold and snowy in winter to stick to your resolution to exercise daily, at least outdoors. In southern Arizona, summer heat reaches 110° or higher for days or weeks at a time. Rain can interfere with an exercise program anywhere. What to do?

Enclosed shopping malls are the answer in cities large enough to have them. Many of them open early for walkers. In smaller towns the community may offer opportunities to use gyms at schools or organizations such as the YMCA. *Just do it!*

How to Maintain Your Weight After Losing—
And Other Important Matters

You have gotten out of the *obese* category if you were there. You have even emerged from the *overweight* category. Then you realized that, even in the *healthy weight* range, you still had some extra weight that kept you from achieving the appearance and feeling you really want. So you have eliminated those excessive pounds also. You look and feel just as you desire.

Maintaining Your Best Weight. What is your best weight? It is the weight, within the *healthy* range, at which you look and feel as you want to. You have probably revised your weight goal as you were losing successfully. At the weight you *thought* you desired, you may find some extra fat. You can lose it by continuing your weight-losing phase a little longer. I hope that you will not compromise with those last few extra pounds. There is no reason to do so. *You are in charge!*

When you reach your best weight, you will need to exchange your *weight-losing* program for a more liberal *weight-maintaining* program. The exact number of calories to hold a steady weight depends mainly on your height and your physical activity. You don't have to do any calculation, like starting with 30% more calories than your weight-losing program and watching the scales to see whether you are holding your best weight.

The basic rule for not regaining the weight you have lost is very simple: *Never regain the first five pounds!* Continue to weigh weekly for the record. That will always be an important part of your life style if you are to stay slim and trim. If your weight begins to increase, continuing that level of intake is obviously unsuitable. *Don't let that increase in weight reach five pounds— ever!* If you gain even two or three pounds, it is time to return to your weight-losing level of eating. This will reinforce what you already know: *You are totally in charge.* That's what a commitment to weight reduction is—taking charge of the situation and knowing that you have the ability to bring your weight to whatever level you desire and keep it there. You do.

How many times have you heard some one say, "I lost ___ pounds on the _____ Diet? And how many of them have continued to their ideal, slim-trim weight? How many have gone back to their old, fat weights within a year? Does your past experience with "yo-yo" dieting (or just reading about it) discourage you from pursuing the successful program of my book? It shouldn't.

I would be disappointed if anyone were ever to call this simple, sound, basic plan for weight control "The Parsons Diet." When your friends commend you on losing excessive pounds and ask how you have achieved (or are achieving) your goal, please say, "I just decided to take charge of my life, learn calories and some simple strategies for controlling them. Then I did it."

Mention the book, of course, and recommend it. But there is no "Parsons Diet." My goal is just to teach basic principles. You have always understood how your bank balance works. Now you know that your weight works the same way, and you will make sure to take out more than you put in.

Phil McGraw, PhD (TV's popular "Dr. Phil") says he overheard some one comment on his approach, "What he says is just common sense." To which, Dr. Phil says, "Well, duh!" My approach to the Obesity Epidemic is to declare war on it, one person at a time. Right now you are that person. I would be highly complimented if some one said the same thing about my approach as they did about Dr. McGraw's take on other matters.

Not that Dr. Phil has ignored obesity. How can anyone with a forum like his ignore the Epidemic? He has told some of his very (morbidly) obese guests that they know they are responsible for this predicament, but the important thing is *why* they have eaten themselves into such a situation. He's right, and such people do need professional help with the emotional problems that, by leading to massive obesity, are threatening life (heart attack, stroke) and limb (degenerative joint disease).

However, the vast majority of fat people are just people whose unsuitable (or nonexistent) calorie management has made them obese. As we said at the outset, you *do* have the brains and ability to take charge and work your way back to a slim-trim weight. You got that fat (even if only relatively few pounds—let's say 10 or 20) over a period of time, and you won't lose all of the weight in a short time. However, by applying the correct strategies consistently, day in and day out, you *will* see steady improvement (your weekly weight loss diary) and you *will* achieve your goal.

Let me know. Now what? For one thing, take a minute and let me know of your success, so I won't think that *Tough Talk* is just another entry in the "98% failure" approaches to the problem. Send me the facts, condensed from your weight reduction diary, at Lilac Press, PO Box 1356, Scottsdale, AZ 85252-1356. Make a copy of this book's order page and order four books for your friends and relatives who need them. *We'll send you a fifth book free!* Help spread the word, and ask the others to do the same.

As we said before, we are sensitive to the possibility that giving this book to some one might seem to say, "You are fat. Here's a book." That's why the book's cover assures that *"Tough Talk"* doesn't mean that we are scolding a person for being fat. Instead, it tells you to *get tough* with excess fat and get rid of it.

Let me repeat: To pave the way for your giving a copy of the book to others (and for them to do the same eventually), each copy includes a bookmark that says, "Presented with loving concern, knowing that weight control can prevent heart attack and diabetes, while sparing weight-bearing joints." Then it says "A gift for you from" and has space for you to add your name, possibly with a short personal message. I have mentioned this before and repeat it now because of its importance in helping you and others to spread the word.

What else can you do? Here's a partial list. Let me know if you have other great ideas to get the important message out.

- ◆ Watch for activities spearheaded by government health agencies, resulting from the end-of-2001 *Surgeon General's Call to Action.*

- ◆ Contact your Senators and Congressmen in Washington to advocate a federal law that requires publication of calorie information, as discussed previously. This is the most important single part of the needed attack on the Epidemic of Obesity. (See Appendix A.)

- ◆ Help your community leaders to establish safe and adequate areas for exercise. Become a community leader yourself if you have the ability and energy.

- ◆ Work aggressively to persuade schools to require physical education (gym) from grade school through high school.

- ◆ Lead children into activities that give them an hour of exercise daily. Soccer, tennis, and basketball are among the best. But don't overschedule children! One activity at a time works best.

- ◆ Work with equal energy to get fast foods and machines filled with calorie-rich soft drinks out of schools, even though their sponsors buy band uniforms and other tempting inducements.

- ◆ Help others! For persons to whom you don't give a copy of this book, at least talk to them about it and give them the ordering information. They can obtain their own copies from Lilac Press, along with extra copies earmarked for others they know who need the message.

Beyond this book. As stated at the beginning, this presentation is not intended as a complete discussion of the principles or methods of weight reduction. I have always considered this information important for my patients who want to lose weight. Over the years, I have discussed these matters with many patients, dating to my days at the Mayo Clinic (Rochester, Minnesota) and at the Jackson Clinic (Madison, Wisconsin). This written version brings this approach up to date, as it relates to the Epidemic of Obesity, outlined so well by Surgeon General David Satcher at the end of his term. We hope the information will help you to take charge of your life and lose your excessive weight, as it helped many patients during my several decades of office practice.

Other recommended reading. Of course, by now you have your own copy of Allan Borushek's calorie counter (*The Doctor's Pocket Calorie, Fat & Carbohydrate Counter*) and have been using it to help you follow the rule: Never eat an uncounted calorie. Know the calories in everything you eat and set limits.

Ellyn Satter, formerly an associate of mine at the Jackson Clinic, has degrees as a registered dietitian (RD) and in psycho-therapy (emphasizing eating disorders). You can learn more about Ellyn and her work at her web site: **www.ellynsatter.com**

She has written several books. The two I have are truly delightful. *Secrets of Feeding a Healthy Family* teaches readers not to be afraid of food and how to enjoy food and cooking, with the family in mind. As she summarizes her philosophy: "The secret of feeding a healthy family is threefold: love good food, trust yourself, and teach your children to do the same." This is a great book for the reader in charge of feeding the family.

Child of Mine details Ellyn's philosophy of feeding a child from birth through pre-school years, with many words of wisdom, including letting your child be a child. As soon as I had paged through my copy, I gave it to my daughter, who had recently emerged from the *Feeding Your Toddler (12 to 36 Months)* stage to *Feeding Your Pre-Schooler* with her son.

I recommend both of these books to anyone who wants to read more along these lines. You can order them at your bookstore.

If ever you decide you don't want to buy a book that the bookstore orders for you (these, or my *Cholesterol Control Without Diet! The Niacin Solution*), they won't mind. They'll just put your copy on the shelf—which is what Ellyn and I wanted all along. We would also like our books on the shelves of your public library. You can help by calling the library and requesting that they put these books (including the one you are reading) into their collection.

A Few Final Thoughts—
And a Last-minute Surprise

About You—and Others. Several times we have said, as you have been reading, that the only statistic that really matters is one person—you. By learning the book's lessons and using them consistently, you *will* succeed in losing your excess fat. By continuing to monitor your weight once a week and making sure you never regain the first five pounds, you *will* maintain that ideal weight. You will continue a regular exercise program to keep that fitness level for the rest of your life.

Be proud that, by your own effort and dedication, you have stepped out of the Obesity Epidemic. Can you help others to make this important step? You can. Start with family members and friends who have extra fat. Then be sure to help to prevent others from becoming overweight or obese—especially young persons.

Must you share this life-saving and life-improving information with others? Not really, if you absolutely want to keep it to yourself. But people will notice your success, compliment you and ask how you have achieved it. You *will* share the source of your information, won't you? To make this easier, you could make copies of the order page (page 136). Carry them with you, and hand one to each person who expresses interest.

We hope that many readers will join us in attacking the Epidemic by buying four copies of the book (and receiving a fifth book free). When you give them to those relatives, friends, and co-workers, please ask each of them, in turn, to give copies to five persons who need the book's help. Then ask that group to give copies to five others—and on and on.

A Last-Minute Surprise. As I was putting finishing touches on this book (early 2003), my favorite political discussion program brought me a pleasant surprise. Host-coordinator John McLaughlin closed his weekly *The McLaughlin Group* (PBS) with a news item about obesity. Opening by labeling Maine "the most obese state" in a recent poll, he went on to list several measures that the Maine legislature had passed. He read his lead-in remarks over a series of video clips, showing a series of fat shapes that could have been filmed in any state of the Union.

The new Maine laws require fast food places to furnish "nutritional information" about their foods. [My reaction: All that matters is *calories*. Don't burden people with irrelevant information that just complicates the public's thinking, possibly obscuring the important message.] Another measure was designed to keep fast foods and calorie-rich soft drinks out of schools. Still another provision encouraged more multi-use paths for exercise.

As you know, I have encouraged you to be an activist. The labeling of all food ads in all media, all menus, cooking shows and cooking segments, recipe columns, and the like *can and should be legislated at the federal level.* Why fight the battle 50 times in 50 states, only to come up with a series of un-even laws that may or may not educate everyone about calories?

Appendix A is a sample letter you can adapt to contact your two Senators and one Representative. Please urge your friends to do so as well. Newspaper editors can further the cause immeasurably with editorials that encourage their readers to join the effort. Why not write a letter to the editor, mentioning our goal and the book? I'll do what I can on talk shows across the nation, including reiterating this plea to foster federal legislation.

Initially this book will be available only by mail order from Lilac Press. That's because we have set the price so low ($9.95 US) that we can't afford to give the book to wholesalers, who take a 55% discount, allowing them make a profit when they sell to bookstores. Starting with a small first printing to test the waters, we will seek sponsors for what needs to be done: Print larger numbers of books. Write and publish a smaller, simplified version. Translate both versions into Spanish. Get both versions into the hands of those who don't buy and read books. Enlist employers, service organizations, doctors, educators. In short: Spread the word! Can we do it? *Yes, we can!* You lead the way!

Appendix A

You can adapt this sample letter to meet your needs in asking your two Senators and one Congressman to sponsor a "Truth in Calories" bill. You can get their addresses from your newspaper. Mine goes to Arizona's junior Senator, Jon Kyl:

(Date, name & address of lawmaker)

Dear Senator Kyl:

The Epidemic of Obesity in the USA is a matter of record and is apparent to anyone who looks around in public places. Before leaving his post, former Surgeon General David Satcher documented the Epidemic in *The Surgeon General's Call to Action to Prevent and Decrease Overweight and Obesity 2001.* So far our government has done little to implement its recommendations.

A new book, *Tough Talk About Fat! How to Reach and Maintain Your Ideal Weight* tackles the problem with readable, no-nonsense teaching that urges the reader to *get tough* and lose excess weight. *It recommends federal legislation* compelling not only fast food chains, but all restaurants, TV cooking programs and cooking segments, newspaper recipes, and food ads in all media *to show prominently the number of calories* in their products.

[Choose one of the next two sentences.—WBP] A copy of the book is enclosed. [OR] A copy of the chapter that advises this legislation (pages 69-74) is enclosed. The principles of such legislation are on pages 70-72, titled *Getting Tough with Food Advertising.* This is analogous to banning tobacco advertising on TV. Obesity is passing up smoking as the leading cause of preventable deaths in the US.

The author emphasizes that weight control is like your bank balance, going up or down as you put in more than you take out, and *vice versa.* He urges the reader to know the calories in all foods he eats, especially those eaten frequently. In a chapter on fast foods and pizza (pages 51-60), he examines their caloric contents and reaches the conclusion that there is no low-calorie fast food or pizza. *Revealing calorie totals across the board* will be an important step toward helping the public with calorie control.

The author points out that by reducing your current intake by 500 calories a day, you will lose a pound a week, when the total deficit reaches 3500 calories. If you reduce your daily intake by 700 (not hard to do if you have had a couple beers or drinks a day, snacks, desserts, candy), you will lose a pound every five days. So one can just trim last week's eating habits and lose four to six pounds a month without counting another calorie!

A TV ad should show, in easy-to-read numbers, the calories for a Big Mac (590), medium fries (540), or BK Double Whopper with Cheese (1020). Not acceptable when your daily target is 1200-1500 calories, is it? Here's where such numbers would be required:

- Fast food ads & menus
- All restaurant menus, buffets, cafeterias
- Food ads in all media, except grocery ads for foods
- TV cooking shows or cooking segments
- Recipe columns in newspapers and magazines
- School cafeterias
- Bars, as well as beer and liquor ads

Please do the American public a favor by sponsoring a bill that will accomplish this purpose. This could lead to competition among food purveyors to popularize low-calorie fare to combat the Epidemic, as the Surgeon General hoped.

Tough Talk About Fat! is currently available only from the publisher, Lilac Press. If you want your staff to research this, details can be found on the publisher's web site, www.cholesterolnodiet.com, including ordering information.

By enlisting your colleagues' help, you can be instrumental in preventing heart attacks, diabetes, and premature deaths, while sparing weight-bearing joints. Thank you for taking this important step toward fighting the Epidemic of Obesity that is overtaking our society.

INDEX

ABOUT THE AUTHOR

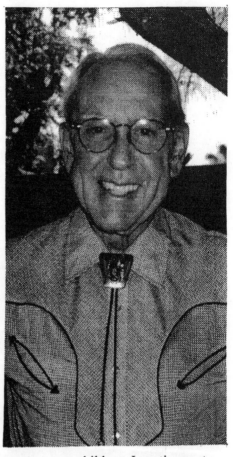

Dr. Bill Parsons was born in Apollo, Pennsylvania and raised in Pittsburgh, where he had his pre-medical and medical education at the University of Pittsburgh. During his training in internal medicine at the Mayo Clinic, he learned from Canadian doctors that large doses of niacin could reduce cholesterol. After conducting the first systematic study of the drug's effect, he went on to pioneer its clinical use and, with his Mayo colleagues, report niacin's success to the medical world. A charter member of the Council of Arteriosclerosis of the American Heart Association, he has written chapters on niacin's use in several books, as well as many articles in medical journals.

After practicing internal medicine for 18 years in Madison, Wisconsin, where he continued his niacin research, and for 21 years in Scottsdale, Arizona, he retired late in 1999.

Bill and his wife, Lynn, have two grown children. In retirement he enjoys playing tennis, doing talk show interviews about his books, and relaxing in their cabin on the Mogollon Rim, near the White Mountains of Arizona.

In addition to *Tough Talk About Fat! How to Reach and Maintain Your Ideal Weight*, Bill is the author of *Cholesterol Control Without Diet! The Niacin Solution*. Its hardcover first edition was succeeded by an updated, expanded second edition (paperback, 2003). Both books are written for the general public. Doctors enjoy them also and recommend them to their patients.

GIVE
Tough Talk About Fat!
How to Reach and Maintain Your Ideal Weight
TO YOUR <u>DOCTOR</u>, <u>FRIENDS</u>, <u>LOVED ONES</u>

THIS BOOK CAN ONLY BE ORDERED FROM
Lilac Press
P.O. Box 1356
Scottsdale, AZ 85252-1356

❑ **YES,** I want ____ copies of *Tough Talk About Fat! How to Reach and Maintain Your Ideal Weight* at $9.95 each, plus $4.00 shipping (for total order).

    Arizona residents please add $0.71 sales tax per book
    Canadian orders need a postal money order in US funds.

HERE'S A SPECIAL OPPORTUNITY:

❑ **SEND ME 4 COPIES** of *Tough Talk About Fat! How to Reach and Maintain Your Ideal Weight* for a total of $39.80, plus $5.00 shipping (entire order). *I will receive a 5th copy free!* (Arizona and Canadian provisions as above.)

AND WHILE WE'RE ON THE SUBJECT:

❑ **I WANT** ____ copies of *Cholesterol Control Without Diet! The Niacin Solution* (2nd edition, 2003) at $14.95 each, plus $4.00 shipping (entire order).
    (Arizona and Canadian provisions as above.)

❑ **SEND ONE COPY OF EACH OF THE ABOVE BOOKS** for $22.00 total, plus $4.00 shipping.
    (Arizona and Canadian provisions as above.)

Name_____

Address_____

City/State/Zip_____

Phone_____ Please make your check payable to **Lilac Press**

136